P9-DIG-234

DATE DUE

DEMCO, INC. 38-2931

MY PROSTATE AND ME

RC
280
.P7
M37
1994

MY PROSTATE AND ME

Dealing with Prostate Cancer

WILLIAM MARTIN

AFTERWORD BY
PETER T. SCARDINO, M.D.
DIRECTOR, MATSUNAGA-CONTE PROSTATE CANCER
RESEARCH CENTER, BAYLOR COLLEGE OF MEDICINE
CHAIRMAN, PROSTATE HEALTH COUNCIL OF THE
AMERICAN FOUNDATION OF UROLOGIC DISEASE

CADELL & DAVIES
NEW YORK

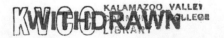
KALAMAZOO VALLEY
WITHDRAWN COLLEGE
LIBRARY

APR 0 6 1995

Cadell & Davies™

An imprint of Multi Media Communicators, Inc.
575 Madison Avenue, Suite 1006
New York, NY 10022

Copyright © 1994 by William Martin. All rights reserved. This book, or parts thereof, may not be reproduced in any form or by any means without written permission from the publisher. For information address: Cadell & Davies.

Cadell & Davies™ is a trademark of Multi Media Communicators, Inc.

Cover design by Jim Hellman and Tim Ladwig
Cover photo of William Martin by Lawrence Hitz

ISBN: 1-56977-888-4

Library of Congress...

10 9 8 7 6 5 4 3 2 1

Printed in the United States of America

To,
in order of appearance,

J. David Bybee, M.D.
C. Eugene Carlton, Jr., M.D.
Richard J. Babaian, M.D.
Patrick C. Walsh, M.D.
Pat Meyers, R.N.
Peter T. Scardino, M.D.
Alejandro L. Rosas, M.D.

—Healers

Samantha
Jenna
Molly
Laura

—Inspiration

With special thanks to
Carolyn Schum and Irene Albright

CONTENTS

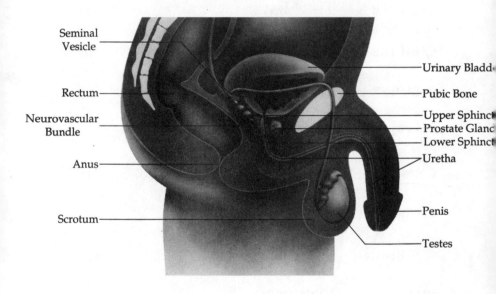

Seminal
Vesicle

Rectum

Neurovascular
Bundle

Anus

Scrotum

Urinary Bladd

Pubic Bone

Upper Sphinc

Prostate Glanc

Lower Sphinct

Uretha

Penis

Testes

CHAPTER 1

My Walnut

My prostate and I were not exactly strangers. At first, I hardly noticed its enlarged role in my life. I had always drunk large quantities of liquids, with the consequent need for frequent trips to the rest room. But about ten years ago, when I was still in my mid-forties, the interval between trips began to grow shorter and the urgency a bit more pressing. I was aware that this was a common side effect of aging, without knowing precisely why, and managed to take it with some good humor. Around the time I turned fifty, a birthday that has a way of impressing one with the fact that the road ahead is likely to be shorter than the one behind, I typically responded to how-does-it-feel-to-be-fifty questions by saying that although my sight and memory were fading, I could pee more often than ever, even at night, when younger men were sleeping. Inevitably, the laughter broke clearly along age lines, with men over fifty in the lead, followed closely by their wives.

Not long afterward, in the course of a regular physical examination, my internist, David Bybee, asked, as part of a long series of questions, if I was

1

noticing any changes in my pattern of urination, such as greater frequency, having to get up one or more times during the night, difficulty in starting, diminished stream, a sensation of not quite finishing, or occasional dribbling. I registered a perfect score. He then performed that highlight of every middle-aged man's physical, the digital rectal examination, identified in urological literature simply as a DRE.

Most men do not enjoy this part of their visit to the doctor. Some, in fact, decline their physician's offer to perform a DRE. I tend to accept official procedures without much resistance and acceded to Dr. Bybee's request that I drop my trousers and bend over, facing away. In addition to being my primary physician, he is also my friend, so I was relatively relaxed. He inserted a gloved and well-lubricated finger into my rectum and began to feel, quite diligently, my prostate gland. I grimaced, my eyes watered, and I hoped he would hurry. Finally, after a long twenty or thirty seconds, he removed his finger, stripped off his glove, and gave me a brief lesson in anatomy.

The prostate gland, he explained, is attached to the base of the bladder, in front of the rectum. At orgasm and ejaculation, it produces the fluid that carries the sperm (produced by the testes) through the penis to whatever happens to be waiting for it nearby. This mingling of substances takes place in the urethra, a tube that runs right through the prostate on its way from the bladder to the end of the penis. That little bit of plumbing is the problem. In a perfectly healthy gland, which is about the size of a walnut, the urethra has plenty of room to perform its small repertoire of tasks. When the prostate starts to grow, however, as it does in most middle-aged men, it typically constricts the urethra, creating some or all of the symptoms to which I had just confessed. This condition has a name: benign prostate hyperplasia (or hypertrophy) or, more simply, BPH. My growth, he said, was a little larger than normal for my age—the *plasia* was more *hyper* than he had expected—but nothing to be too concerned about. As its name indicates, BPH is benign. It isn't cancer and it doesn't turn into cancer. If the gland were cancerous, he explained, he would probably be able to feel a lump or a ridge or some other kind of hardness or irregularity. He had felt nothing unusual other than the enlargement. He would keep an eye on it, so to speak, and if my symptoms got worse, we could talk about what to do then.

I wasn't worried. My symptoms weren't extreme, and I knew that treatment existed, though I was not clear about details. I remembered that my father, when he was about 70, had undergone a surgical procedure known popularly as "a Roto-Rooter job," and that he had pronounced it a great

success. On the second day of his recovery, he
boasted that he "could pee over a ten-wire fence"
and allowed that, had he known about this operation, he would have had it done years earlier.
Now, I knew about it years earlier than he had,
and I would be ready when the time came.

With the exception of some common allergies,
which I keep under control with biweekly self-
administered injections, and stomach pains that
strike in times of stress, I have enjoyed almost perfect health throughout my adult life. In my first
twenty-five years of teaching at Rice University, I
missed class only three times because of illness.
Given that record, I have often stretched the time
between physical exams longer than perhaps I
should have, and an unbroken string of satisfactory results on the standard battery of tests had
made me quite complacent. Thus, on the occasion
of my next exam, in 1990, about two years after
the one just described, I was mildly surprised
when David Bybee told me I had scored a bit
higher than normal on a relatively new blood test
he had given me. It was called a PSA, for prostate
specific antigen, and it seemed to be useful in giving an early warning sign that a man might be
developing cancer of the prostate. The normal
range was 0-4. My score was 6.4. (I would later
learn that this figure reflects nanograms, or bil-
lionths of a gram, per milliliter.) Some urologists,

he said, didn't think there was much reason to worry until the score got up to around 12 or so. The test is prostate-specific, but not cancer-specific. An enlarged prostate can raise the score even when no cancer is present, but cancer tissue causes it to zoom upward much more rapidly than does normal tissue. His digital examination had indicated nothing more than slight continued enlargement, but he felt it would be worthwhile for me to have an ultrasonic examination of my prostate, just to play it safe. He could arrange to have it done at the Department of Urology at the Baylor College of Medicine.

I didn't know what such an exam would cost, but I assumed my insurance would pay for most of it and I could afford the rest. I have long taken some comfort in living just five blocks from the Texas Medical Center, with its collection of world-famous hospitals, medical schools, and research institutions. No matter how long a shot it was, it didn't make sense to turn down a chance to use some of that collective expertise to check on the possibility that I might have cancer.

A transrectal ultrasound (TRUS) is not nearly as much fun as a DRE. After removing my trousers, I crawled up on a table and lay on my side while the technician operated the machine and discussed what he saw with a young urology resident. Though it is sonic rather than optical, the sensation is rather like having a TV camera—with knobs removed—poked into one's rectum and aimed here and there for ten or fifteen minutes, producing shadowy images on a little Sony monitor that I was invited to watch. Having never seen anyone's prostate nor, for that matter, an ultrasound image of anything other than a fetus of one of my granddaughters, I couldn't make much of what I saw. The technician said my prostate was more pear-shaped than round, but that this was a normal variation. Other than that, he and the resident saw nothing to indicate the presence of any kind of cancerous growth. Just as I thought.

Not quite a year after that exam, my wife Patricia and I flew to California to visit our son Jeff, his wife Suzanne, and daughters Samantha and Jenna, the latter of whom was brand new. We spent a night in Santa Barbara at that charming "small hotel with a wishing well" where Charlie Chaplin and Fatty Arbuckle used to carouse, I gave a lecture at Pepperdine University, and Jeff showed us around Twentieth-Century Fox studios, where he worked as a writer for "The Simpsons." It was an entirely satisfying interlude. Then, on the last day of our stay, as if contemplating silent movies and watching my grown son pursue a successful career had somehow reminded a sensitive prostate of the rapid passage of time, I was suddenly stricken with the worst urinary discomfort I had ever experienced. The need to urinate was truly burning, voiding brought as much pain as relief, and what relief ensued was dismayingly short-lived. I was relieved that the flight back to Houston was on a DC-10, which enabled me to alternate aisles on my way to the toilet, in an effort not to call attention to the frequency of my trips.

The first night at home, I made eleven trips to the bathroom, about nine more than usual. The next morning, I called Dr. Bybee's office, described my symptoms, and managed to get an afternoon appointment. He listened to my symptoms and performed a DRE that was not only eye-popping but produced a small amount of milky discharge, which he collected on a glass slide. He smiled and rendered his verdict: a classic case of prostatitis. My walnut-sized nemesis had developed an infection. Prostatitis typically occurs in younger men and can bear some relation either to lack of sexual activity or to a sudden burst of activity after a period of abstinence. None of those conditions fit my case, but none were required. Sometimes it just happens, and I clearly had it. Fortunately, it was curable, though not overnight. He prescribed a six-week regimen of an antibiotic especially formulated to penetrate into the prostate, and he invited me to return every few days for a week or two to have my gland hand-milked. He drew blood for another PSA test, just as a precaution. Then, as a parting shot, he suggested that I try to have sex as often as possible. Throw me in the briar patch.

On my next visit a few days later, Dr. Bybee told me my PSA count was up to about 8, approximately 25 percent higher than my previous test. That was not good, but neither was it alarming. Just as enlargement can raise the score, so can prostatitis. My score would probably go down when the infection subsided. I acknowledged my relief at learning that my new intense discomfort was traceable mainly to an infection, but volunteered that the normal state of affairs was no picnic. I asked whether he thought I ought to consider the Roto-Rooter procedure, which a recent consultation with my Modern Home Medical Adviser had taught me to identify as a transurethral resection of the prostate (TURP).

David Bybee is a bright, compassionate, and thoroughly honest man, but he is not what one would describe as earthy. He said, "Oh, I don't think I'd rush into that. One of the things it does is to send the ejaculate back into the bladder, so that your orgasm is dry. And that...well...it might not be as much fun. As long as your symptoms are not bothering you too much, I'd put that off as long as I could. We're both just getting older."

Happily, the prostatitis subsided and disappeared as predicted, but over the next eighteen months, my prostate gradually but perceptibly got a tighter grip on my urethra. I added a trip or two to my nighttime routine, the interval between voidings diminished to less than an hour during the day, and my body's announcement of the need to urinate sometimes came so suddenly and with such intensity that a wait of as little as ten minutes was simply out of the question. I seldom made it through a meeting of any consequence without having to excuse myself at least once. I dared not try to teach on Tuesdays and Thursdays, when classes run 80 minutes, and standing around to talk to students after a 50-minute class was often a major challenge. During the 1992-93 academic year, the Rice sociology department sponsored a series of public lectures on urban issues. As one of the organizers of the series, it often fell to me to introduce the speaker and to sit either on the dais or the front row. Without exception, the question-and-answer session following the speeches provided my bladder with a severe test. On more than half of those occasions, I had to leave my seat and walk the length of the auditorium to reach a rest room, typically returning just in time to bring the evening to a close. I could joke with myself that "I'm a big guy with a big prostate," but it really wasn't much fun.

Increasingly, strategic planning for urination became a conscious part of my routine. I learned to void just before leaving the house and then again upon arriving at almost any destination—church, a restaurant, my office, a friend's home—in the hope, often vain, that I would not have to excuse myself more than once during an average sojourn. At a concert or theater, I tried to arrange for seats on the aisle, and at intermission I tried to use a closed stall rather than a urinal, to avoid having some young man in line behind me ask if he could "play through." At public gatherings, I ignored requests to move toward the center. At movies, I learned that episodes of high excitement or intense emotion are typically followed by slow spots that allow a quick trip to the toilet. (Scenes beginning with a shot of a car or bus on a long, straight highway are ideal.) I began to select supermarkets and video stores less for their stock and prices than for their provision of public rest rooms, though I quickly learned that one can find an unadvertised rest room in most grocery stores simply by walking through the swinging doors next to the meat counter.

Eventually, I learned the location of the john in virtually all the places I frequented. At the Brazos Bookstore near the university, you go straight back through the open door at the rear of the display area. In the sprawling Bookstop at Alabama and Shepherd, the rest rooms are locked, but the key is attached to a whiskbroom right next to the cash register. You don't have to ask for it; just take it. And in the River Oaks Book Shop, you are welcome to use the small unisex bathroom upstairs in the children's section, but the ladies who run the store appreciate it if male customers heed a sign asking them not to rest their hands on the wall over the toilet. (It's a balancing feat that takes some getting used to, but it can be learned.)

Travel called for similar calculation and logistic expertise. On most weekends, Patricia and I make a three-hour drive between Houston and Wimberley, a little town in the Texas Hill Country where we have a home to which we expect eventually to retire. If the westbound traffic on a Friday afternoon was especially heavy, we would need to stop at the Knox Truck Stop near Sealy. I like that one both because the coffee is good and because, if I don't want coffee, the rest room is far enough from the cash register that the cashier is not likely to notice that I didn't buy anything, or perhaps she might think I just dropped in to pick up an assortment of exotic condoms. On a light-traffic and low-liquid day, I could sometimes last the 70 minutes it takes to make it to Columbus, where McDonald's Golden Arches welcome the squirming traveler.

Just a few miles past Columbus sits a roadside

rest area whose purpose is quite explicit and the accommodations acceptable, if one doesn't mind standing in a quarter-inch of water of indeterminate origin. Further down the road, Grumpy's at Flatonia and Love's at Luling offer additional shame-free opportunities for relief and the chance to refill our no-spill insulated coffee mugs. In case you are wondering, I am quite aware of the connection between caffeine and bladder stimulation, but compromise has its role in a life of moderation, and I seldom drink more than two cups a day anyway.

I should make it clear that we never stopped at all these places on the same trip. On the other hand, we almost never stopped less than twice during the first two hours. The last hour of the journey offers fewer opportunities for convenient relief, but by that time I was usually fairly well drained. In case of extreme need, we could sometimes find a country road to turn down or, in a real pinch, there was always the empty Snapple bottle under the seat. In general, my condition made me feel mildly rueful rather than genuinely humiliated, and Patricia laughed with me rather than at me, as best I could determine. If David Bybee thought it best, I could doubtless stand it a while longer, but I could not help pondering whether a dry orgasm might not be less discomfiting than a chronically constricted urethra.

Despite intensifying symptoms, I did not see Dr. Bybee professionally again until the summer of 1993, when I had my next general physical. As usual, I went in several days before my appointment to let his nurses draw blood, collect a urine sample, and run an EKG. When he examined me directly, I told him my urinary symptoms had worsened and he told me my PSA count was up to 8.23. Apparently, prostatitis had not been the sole culprit for the higher reading the previous year. He thought I needed another ultrasound. He also thought it was time to try some medication. He talked about Hytrin, an "alpha-blocker" developed to control mild high blood pressure but known to be useful in relaxing the bladder and urethra sufficiently to relieve some of the symptoms of BPH. It wouldn't affect the size of my prostate, but it might moderate my discomfort. The other choice was Proscar, a highly touted drug developed by Merck and designed actually to shrink the prostate. The main and relatively uncommon side effect documented so far is diminution of libido, or sex drive.

I knew about Proscar. Merck has long been a favorite stock of mine and I had raised my holdings a bit when the new drug was introduced. Unfortunately, I held on a bit too long after President Clinton began attacking the pharmaceutical companies, but I had read a good bit about the drug and had decided that loss of libido was, at this point, too great a price to pay for a smaller prostate, especially since the drug has proved effective in only about half the men who take it. I agreed to give Hytrin a try. The main possible side effects were drowsiness or dizziness, particularly in people with low blood pressure. Since my usual pressure is around 115 over 70 (normal, as most people know, is 120 over 80), he suggested I build up my tolerance slowly and take the drug just before going to bed, to minimize any dizziness or drowsiness. Finally, he asked me to come back for another PSA test in two or three weeks, since considerable fluctuation is possible, and to plan on yet another visit in sixty days, to see if the Hytrin was having any effect.

As I had fully expected, the ultrasound showed nothing irregular. My insurance company and I were out $280, and I was still as healthy as ever, except for my engorged gland. Even better, the Hytrin seemed to be working. It was hard to be certain, but the calls of nature, while still fairly frequent, did seem somewhat less demanding. A couple of times, I slept through the night without having to go to the bathroom even once. About that same time, a widely advertised national screening program for prostate cancer prompted thousands of men to show up at clinics to have doctors probe their rectums and draw their blood.

For once, I felt ahead of the curve on the latest biomedical fad. I had already been there, done that,
received a clean bill of health, and had some little
pills that were fixing me up. When I got a mail
order solicitation to buy a vitamin and mineral
supplement called Prostata, which the flier
assured me would shrink my prostate, lower my
PSA, and add zip to my sex life, I ordered a two-
month supply. They couldn't make claims like
that if they weren't true, could they? I was on a
roll.

Then I got a letter and a follow-up call from
David Bybee. My sixty days weren't up yet, but
my score on the second PSA test had been 8.02.
That was down a little from the 8.23, but still high
enough to be worrisome. He thought I ought to
see a specialist and gave me the name of
C. Eugene Carlton, who was, he noted, the former
chair of the Department of Urology at Baylor and
the incoming president of the American
Urological Association. Gene Carlton, he said, is
not overly aggressive in his approach, but might
well suggest I have a biopsy done on my prostate.
In his matter-of-fact way, he explained that the
biopsy would involve drawing tissue samples by
means of a spring-loaded gun inserted through
the rectum. It might hurt a bit for a couple of
hours and there would probably be some blood in
my urine and ejaculate for several days. There

was also the possibility of an abscess, but that didn't happen too often.

Nothing about that description sounded appealing to me and I did not rush to contact Dr. Carlton. To slow things down further, school was just starting and I was having to prepare class materials and attend the usual round of meetings. Then, two chance conversations moved me to action. At an informal dinner for a small group of my freshman advisees, I fell into conversation with an alumnus who was hosting the event and who happens to be a urologist. I mentioned that I had been giving urology a great deal of thought in recent weeks, and he asked if I knew my PSA count. When I told him it was an 8, his expression clearly indicated he regarded that news rather seriously. I told him I had had two ultrasounds and both had been negative, but he said, "Still, that's pretty high. You ought to have your doctor watch that."

A few days later, I was having lunch with Frank, a friend about fifteen years older than I. We got to discussing the President's healthcare proposals and I ventured that, while I favored some kind of general program, I feared it would be difficult to keep the costs from becoming ruinous. I volunteered that my doctor, whom I trust and admire, had just prescribed an ultrasonic exam of my prostate and, even though it had

shown nothing whatever, now thought I should
have it biopsied. I knew his concern was primarily for me and that he was not prescribing tests to
fatten his or a colleague's bank account, but I also
felt fairly sure I was being overtreated. I could
afford it, so I would do it, but I wasn't convinced
it was necessary and I could see that sort of thing
happening millions of times over in a govern-
ment-sponsored program, even if all the physicians in the country were as conscientious and
ethical as mine. My friend said, "Well, I know
how you feel. Last spring, my doctor got worried
about my PSA count and sent me to a urologist.
He referred me to M. D. Anderson.* They did a
biopsy and drew samples from six areas. I went
downstairs to the cafeteria and had a cup of cof
fee. I felt great and I had no worries at all. When
I came back up in about fifteen minutes, the doctor told me that three of the six samples contained
cancer. I was floored."

"If you don't mind my asking," I didn't mind
asking, "what was your PSA count?"

"It had bounced around. At first, it was 6, then
7, then 5, then 8."

"Hmm. What did they do?"

"At M. D. Anderson, they do a lot with radiation, which was fine with me. My brother had a

*The University of Texas M.D. Anderson Cancer
Center in Houston.

prostatectomy two years ago, and he didn't bounce back. That is a mean, cruel operation. But let's face it. Doctors—surgeons especially—want you to get well, but they are also in a business, and they are going to do what makes the money. But what they did with me at Anderson was just the easiest thing you could imagine. I went in five days a week for six weeks for a radiation treatment. After the first visit, when they got everything lined up just right and marked me up, it only took about fifteen minutes from start to finish. Toward the end, I would get a little tired in the late afternoon, but that was the only thing I ever noticed. That was just the happiest, most upbeat place I have ever been in. It was such a pleasant experience that I almost think a person ought to go through it whether he needed it or not."

Frank, as you might gather, is man with a positive outlook. I do not hold that against him, but I might have paid less attention had he not told me that a PSA count similar to mine had corresponded to cancer in half his tissue samples. I called Gene Carlton's office that afternoon and set up an appointment for the following week.

CHAPTER 2

THE NEWS

University professors can fool themselves about their position in the life cycle. The clientele never ages, young colleagues tend to treat their elders as peers, and the constant presence of youthful activities and attitudes can lull one into overlooking the inexorable march of maturity. A visit to a urology clinic can dispel that illusion rather quickly. The Scott Department of Urology at the Baylor College of Medicine, just across the street from Rice, is one of the finest in the world, with a stellar roster of researchers and practitioners, but its patients are mostly old guys who are having trouble peeing. As I walked in, I met David Bybee coming out. Since he is affiliated with Baylor, I assumed he was consulting with one of the clinicians about something, but apparently he was there as a patient. He greeted me and smiled, observing with a chuckle that "This is where the old men meet." That much was unmistakable. The average age of the dozen or so men waiting to see their physician must have been in the high sixties. None looked cheerful; some looked desperately ill.

Two or three were accompanied by their wives. I assumed that was a bad sign.

Clinics associated with medical schools and research hospitals can be excellent places to obtain high-quality care, but one needs to understand that appointment times are intended as approximations. By the time Dr. Carlton's nurse called my name, I was beginning to experience a familiar discomfort. A sign in the waiting room instructed patients who needed to urinate to speak to a nurse first. I assumed this was because the doctor might want a urine sample and resolved to wait a few more minutes, but as I sat in the examination room, looking at full-color charts of diseased prostates while waiting for Dr. Carlton to appear, I decided I needed some relief. I disliked seeming over-anxious and having to ask for permission to pee, but I recognized that nurses in a urology clinic would not find my request out of line. Carlton's nurse, Janet Fuentes, is a pert and cheerful Englishwoman who ushered patients in and out in an upbeat and immensely likable manner. When I sought her out and told her of my need, she understood completely, leading me to a little rest room a few feet away, pointing to an odd device that looked like a giant funnel, and instructing me to "just nip it right in there." I was a bit puzzled, since I could easily have hit either a specimen jar or a regulation toilet, but I was in no mood to argue. I did as told and returned to the examination room.

After another short wait, Dr. Carlton appeared, wearing green surgical scrubs and leather moccasins, one of my own favorite casual outfits. I guessed him to be in his late fifties or early sixties. His manner was friendly and straightforward, with no trace of condescension. I felt I was in good hands. We discussed my symptoms, my PSA score, and my unimpressive urine flow rate, which he had just obtained from the magic funnel, for a fee of $95. The last time I used a pay toilet, it cost only two francs. Nothing pointed to sure trouble, but all the signs were a bit unusual for a man my age. "It's not likely, but you could have some cancer in there," he said. "I think you ought to have a biopsy. We can do it right now if you have time."

I agreed, but asked what were the chances of finding cancer. "Eighteen percent," he said. I frowned. I would not consider playing Russian Roulette, and these were worse odds. He picked it up quickly: "Look at it this way: there's an 82-percent chance we won't find anything. Let's see...this is Thursday. Call anytime Monday morning and we'll have the results." Since two ultrasounds had found me clean, I decided to look at the bright side and truly felt little trepidation as he took me to the lab and introduced me to the technician. I thanked him for his help and, quite frankly, figured I might not see him again.

The room and initial procedures were identical to the other ultrasounds I had experienced, one just a few weeks before, so I felt familiar, if not comfortable, with the routine. After poking around with the probe for a while, the technician explained that he was going to extract samples of tissue from selected sections of my prostate with a spring-loaded hollow needle inserted through a tube in the probe. He would tell me just before he pulled the trigger and I would be able to see it at work on the screen. As I contemplated the prospect of having a spring-driven needle zipping through my gland, the technician explained that he would insert the needle slowly; when the spring retracted, the razor-sharp hollow needle would take with it a tiny sample of tissue. That sounded slightly better. Curious, I asked, "Will I feel anything?"

"Oh, yeah," he said, with an inflection that left no doubt. Then, to prove his point, he maneuvered his way into a likely spot and instructed me to take a deep breath. On the screen, I saw the grainy image of a pointed object penetrating my prostate. Deep in my body, I could tell the image was not a mirage. Then, "Thwunk!" The spring sprang and I saw a line of tissue instantaneously disappear. It was not pleasant, but neither was it terrible. I could handle this. Five more times I held my breath and surrendered small parts of myself to science. When it was over, I dressed and waited until the samples could be sealed in little containers and stapled into a paper sack that I took to the pathology lab at Methodist Hospital across the street.

A few months earlier, a "Prime Time Live" segment had criticized Methodist Hospital as unusually luxurious for a non-profit institution. It is easy to get that impression. When I approached the area to which I had been directed, an attractive young woman in a crisp hotel-style uniform stepped forth to ask if she could be of assistance. I told her the nature of my errand and she directed me to a cubicle where a precise young man named Rodney collected some data about me that would help the hospital stay even, if not make a profit. Then I deposited my little sack at a window down the hall and went back to work.

It was nearly 5:00 by the time I got back to the office, and two of my colleagues, Steve and Chad, were taking care of some closing-time tasks in the large general-purpose room outside our individual offices. When I sat down at a computer attached to our laser printer, they noticed I was moving rather gingerly and listing to one side. I explained about the biopsy and observed that it had not been great fun. I told them of my doctor's concern and mentioned the 18-percent odds. We have worked together for more than 20 years, we are all in our fifties, and we are sufficiently aware of our mortality to recognize that someday, bad things would start to happen. But that would be later, much later, not now when we were all in our prime, with children out of college and marriages happy and careers going well. So they, like me, were appropriately troubled but chose to look on the sunny side of the percentages.

As David Bybee had indicated, I felt some discomfort for a couple of hours, but it wasn't serious and it passed. Unfortunately, pain wasn't all that passed. For several days, urination usually began with a spurt of blood, unnerving even when expected. My ejaculate was even bloodier, and orgasm felt strange, as if my prostate was using the occasion to combine pleasure with throwing out the trash.

The next few days were peculiar ones. Because Rice was taking a two-day fall break, Patricia and I had planned a trip to Los Angeles to visit Jeff and his family and to watch the taping of a new sitcom he and his wife Suzanne and a friend of theirs had created. Jeff's career has been a great source of pleasure and pride for us. We had seen the pilot and liked it, and we had looked forward to visiting the Disney Studios, where the show was being produced for NBC. Since it would not

debut until after the first of the year, it was fun to
feel we were in on the early stages of something
he had been pointing toward since he was about
fifteen years old. Now, a slight shadow hovered
over the visit, but it covered only eighteen percent
of our emotional sky and we resolved not to mention it until we could share what we assumed
would be Monday's good news.

One of the treasures of our lives is that we genuinely like, as well as love, our three adult children and their spouses. That makes visits easy.
And, of course, we adore getting to see our granddaughters, of whom there are four at last count.
Suzanne was busy polishing a script she had written, so Jeff served as primary host. On Saturday
afternoon he and I dropped by for a look at Aimee
Semple McPherson's famed Angelus Temple near
Echo Park, then drove past other show-business
landmarks such as the house where Marilyn
Monroe died and Joan Crawford's mansion,
where wire coat hangers were unwelcome. After
lunch on Sunday, he and Patricia and I took
Samantha and Jenna to Disneyland. Though both
girls had been to the park many times, we got to
play the full grandparental role: watching with
delight as they laughed at the Country Bear
Jamboree, checking to see if they were scared during the Pirates of the Caribbean ride, snapping an

excess of pictures as they hugged Mickey, and recalling when it came time to leave that these were not the first children to wail that "We were just starting to have fun." Except when I had to ferret out rest rooms every hour or so, I didn't think much about prostates.

On Monday, everyone went back to work, school, or day care, so Patricia and I drove down the coast toward Laguna Beach, with no particular destination in mind. Around mid-morning, we stopped at a little coffee shop near the ocean at Newport Beach. I had not said anything about the biopsy report, but I had been thinking about it, and had purposely waited until I felt sure there had been time for the lab reports to be delivered. It was now past noon in Houston, so it should be fine. After a walk out on a pier, I stopped at a pay phone and called the clinic. Patricia indicated she had also been thinking it was about time. After I negotiated the automated obstacle course—"If you are a patient, press 'one.'. . . If you wish to speak to your nurse, press 'two.'. . ."—I finally reached a woman named Gwen who, after a bit of checking, told me the results were not available yet. Could I call back in an hour? I was disappointed, since I had wanted to get the good news out of the way so I could enjoy the rest of the day, but I took Gwen at her word.

We drove on down to Emerald Bay, one of the

loveliest spots in the country, and looked at some stunning ocean-front lots, thinking that Jeff and Suzie might enjoy living there someday. Within three weeks, as we watched much of Emerald Bay go up in flames, we decided not to give them too much advice about real estate. For lunch, we stopped at the Ritz-Carlton Hotel on the beach at Dana Point. Nearly two hours had passed, so I made another call. This time, Gwen told me that only Dr. Carlton could give me the results, but that he was with patients in the clinic just now. Could I call back about three?

The report, apparently, was there. I didn't remember Dr. Carlton's exact words, but I was quite sure he had told me his nurse or someone else would be able to give me the results of the biopsy. Why, now, did I have to speak to him?

Lunch was acceptable, with a great view of surfers from an elegant informal dining area overlooking the ocean, but I had trouble keeping my mind on food. As soon as we finished, about 1:00, Patricia and I stepped into one of the large wood-paneled phone booths and rang Houston again. By this time, I not only had the number down cold, but knew the "if-you-wish" codes that would summon a live person. For good or ill, I thought, this time I will find out where I stand. I was too optimistic. "I'm sorry," Gwen reported. "Dr. Carlton has gone home. Let me see if Jan can help you." A long hold. "Mr. Martin, Carolyn is taking Jan's calls this afternoon. I'll try to reach her." Another hold. "I'm sorry. Carolyn doesn't know anything about your tests. Can you call back tomorrow?"

"Will I have to wait until Dr. Carlton comes in?"

"Oh, no. Jan can tell you. I just don't have the report."

By this time, I really didn't care why the swallows come back to Capistrano, but since neither of us had ever been to the famed mission, we gave it a try, checking out the cactus garden, peering in at the actual piano where Leon René wrote the song that made San Juan Capistrano and its swallows famous, and looking at dioramas depicting the conversion of Native Americans by Franciscan friars and the construction of the original mission compound.

I did my duty by all of these sights, but I didn't enjoy them much. Some fear was undoubtedly nibbling around the edges of my psyche, but my more conscious reaction was frustration and irritation at what I took to be bureaucratic incompetence. Gwen had ruined my day, for no good reason. We would all spend Tuesday night at the studio for the taping. For this evening, Monday, I had planned to stop at a deli to pick us some fine little things to snack on when Jeff and Suzie came in from work, and to finish it off with a bottle of champagne to celebrate what I had just found out I didn't have. We'd all be relieved, raise a second glass, and talk about how it had felt to think about cancer—"No, I wasn't really worried, because I had just had the ultrasound, but, of course, there was always a chance, so it was a relief, sure." Then we'd decide what to do for dinner.

Given the fruitless pursuit of information, the champagne and deli treats did not get bought. All that remained was what to do for dinner. Jeff and Suzie, bless their hearts, think of food as fuel, and manage to get remarkable mileage out of low-octane material: frozen pizzas and canned nutritional drinks and pre-sauced pasta wheels scooped out of large plastic bins and zapped in the microwave. By contrast, Patricia and I place food high on the list of sensual pleasures and can recall where we have eaten good meals at moderate prices on virtually every vacation day for the last twenty years. When it became clear that no one else saw any need to grab for more gusto than a plate of day-old sushi could provide, we headed for a little neighborhood Italian restaurant a few blocks away.

Over dinner, I shared my theory with Patricia: If the news had been good, anyone could have given it to me. Since I couldn't reach Dr. Carlton and no one would give it to me, it must be bad. She admitted she could see my point, but thought an alternative hypothesis was just as plausible: Good help is hard to get, and incompetence and insensitivity were just as likely to have been responsible for my frustrating experiences of the day. I decided there was an eighty-two percent chance she was right and turned to more pressing matters. It worked. If more of the world had ready access to properly cooked pasta, well-oiled and thinly sliced garlic, and robust red wine at ten dollars a bottle, Prozac would never have made it to market.

About 8:00 Tuesday morning, when I figured that everyone who needed to come in to the office at Baylor was there, I called once more, with the same frustrating result. Dr. Carlton wouldn't be in until noon, a new voice said, and Jan hadn't come in yet, but as soon as she came in, she could pull my file and would be able to give me the report. Could I call back in a couple of hours?

"Yes," I said, "but let me me get something straight. Yesterday I was told once that only Dr. Carlton could give me the report. Is there any point in my calling back until he comes in?"

"I don't know why anyone told you that," the lady said. "Jan or any of the nurses can give it to you. We just don't have it out right now."

"I don't want to complain," I said, not wanting to complain, "but I am feeling quite frustrated. I was told first that anyone could tell me, then that only Dr. Carlton can tell me, and now once again that anyone can tell me. For two days I have been trying to find out whether I have cancer and I can't get anyone to tell me, when the answer is apparently right inside a manila folder in your office. When someone tells me that only the doctor can give me the news, I can't help but think the news must be bad. That is scary. Do you understand that?"

"I can see why you would feel that way," she said. I listened carefully and noted that she did not insist I was worrying needlessly. She simply reiterated that I should call back in a couple of hours and get the news from Jan or one of the other nurses.

Most sitcoms performed before a live audience have two taping sessions, one in the late afternoon and the other in the early evening. The first is essentially a dress rehearsal, although a well-done scene might make it into the final mix. The afternoon session is usually less tight and, because the audience tends to be older and less receptive to humor that draws heavily on contemporary popular culture, deader. Anxious for us to see their best product, Jeff and Suzanne both encouraged us to pass up that session for the later taping, and to spend the time taking in more L.A. sights. When we dropped Suzanne by the studio, we stepped inside for a few minutes and I slipped into an empty office and made yet another call to Houston. By this time, though disappointed once again, I was hardly surprised to learn that only Dr. Carlton could give me the results of my biopsy, and he would not be in for another hour or so. Could I call back?

Were it not for the fact that I have become accustomed to clerical functionaries who cannot add, subtract, spell, speak grammatically, or answer simple requests without putting me on hold to the accompaniment of "Lite Rock," I would probably have been even more convinced that my darker suspicions about the biopsy were correct. But even with bureaucratic incompetence as an entirely plausible explanation for the run-around I had been getting for two days, the clouds were looming more ominously over my parade.

Because we are now a family with ties to "the business," and also because I like amusement parks, Patricia and I decided to spend the day at Universal Studios. By the time we got our bearings and mapped out a plan of attack, lunch seemed like a good idea, so we dropped into Wolfgang Puck's pizza cafe and ordered a calzone. Assuming that, even at this location, Wolfgang wouldn't be serving microwave fare, I figured I had time to try another call and stepped across the way to a public telephone. This time, I was told that Dr. Carlton was in, but was with a patient. I asked that he be told I was on the phone. It worked.

His voice was cordial, but businesslike. He had delivered news of this sort many times before and appeared to see no point in softening the blow. "Of the six samples we drew," he said, "one, at the base of the gland, showed definite evidence of cancer and two more were pre-cancerous. Something bad is going on in there and we need to take care of it. For a man your age, the thing to do is to take out your prostate. That should give you a ninety percent chance of living a normal life span."

Not totally surprised, I was nonetheless stunned. "What about radiation?" I asked.

"We can do that, but your chances drop to about 70%. I think surgery is the way to go, but it's your choice."

"How soon do I need to decide?"

"There's no great emergency, but I think you ought to do something in a few weeks, not months. I'm going to be out of the office the rest of the week. When you get back into town and check your schedule, make an appointment and we can talk. You're married, aren't you?"

"Yes."

"You'd better bring your wife with you."

That sounded ominous, but I was already

developing a strong desire to hold onto Patricia real tightly, and I didn't imagine that would dissipate entirely by the following week. I told him I would call and said good-bye. I leaned against the wall, swallowed, noticed that something inside my abdomen felt like it had gone into free-fall, and stepped back into a world that would never look quite the same again.

Patricia was facing me as I entered the restaurant, and her expression was one of cautious curiosity. She could tell all was not well.

"Did you get through?"

I nodded.

"What did you find out?"

"I have cancer."

I am aware that worse messages can be delivered and received, but that one is bound to be among the Top Ten pieces of high-impact bad news the average citizen is likely to hear.

I told her what Dr. Carlton had said and that we would be going to see him the following week. We admitted that, even though we had known, intellectually, that this was a possibility, neither of us had really believed it would be true. Numerous negative DREs, three negative ultrasounds, an eighteen percent chance—these did not add up to cancer.

"Oh, Bill," she said, taking my hands as both our eyes started to fill with tears. She told me she loved me more than anything, and I was never more sure that it was both true and my most precious treasure.

Sometime during this conversation, our calzone arrived and, since no one else was at our table, we apparently ate it. After a cup of coffee, Patricia asked, "What do you want to do now?" Nothing was real high on my list, but since we were where we were, I said, "Why don't we go find out how they make movies?" As we left, the waitress told us to have a nice day.

The rest of the afternoon was surreal. It was a kick to see Lt. Columbo's old Peugeot parked by the side of the road, to feel the fire roar through the warehouse set from *Backdraft*, and to bounce around on the *Back to the Future* ride, one of the all-time great illusions. Still, the gnawing heaviness in the pit of my stomach never completely went away, and when we learned there were no more seats for the Wild West shoot-out performance, I was quite content to sit down and curl up with a sixteen-ounce beer. When the time finally came to head back to Disney, I was ready. I'd had about all the excitement I needed for one day.

We arrived at the sound stage just as the first taping session was winding up. Jeff felt the afternoon audience had been even deader than usual and was clearly worried that the episode might not play well in the evening. After an informal

buffet dinner with the cast and crew, he "gave
notes," telling one of the leads to be sure he spoke
the last lines in a scene as clearly as he could without exaggerating, suggesting to a twelve-year-old
actress that she tilt her head a certain way when
she delivered one of her worldly wise comments,
then asking a cameraman to come in a little
tighter on a shot in a pizza parlor. Jeff is the only
one of our children who watched a great deal of
television. It seems to have paid off. He was
sure-handed, tactful, and funny, and it was clear
the folk working with him liked him. We had
watched Jeff show up on skits during his six-year
stint as a writer for David Letterman, and we had
often been able to identify the original provenance
of bits and lines on "The Simpsons," but we had
never seen him in action in charge of his own
show. This was what he had been pointing
toward for years, here it was, and he was clearly
good at it. It was extraordinarily gratifying.

The second taping, before a younger audience,
went much better, and we basked in the positive
things several Disney executives were kind
enough to tell us about Jeff. And I kept thinking
about how much I wanted to be around to see
where all this might lead. My experience as a cancer victim had barely covered eight hours, but I
was already beginning to see the down side.

Because we had to be back at work the next

day, Patricia and I had booked a red-eye flight that left LAX shortly after midnight. On the way to the airport, I sat in the front seat next to Jeff. At the first break in the conversation, I told him I had some bad news. I explained that I had prostate cancer, but that I wasn't going to die, at least not anytime soon, and that our main immediate concern was what to do about it and what effect that would have on our lives.

I knew from experience that acknowledging the mortality of a parent and facing it head-on are two different matters. I could see that Jeff was learning that distinction. His eyes and voice were filling with tears. He put his hand on my knee. "Are you in pain?" he asked.

"No. I feel fine. That's what's so strange."

We talked some more. I don't remember the details, except that he said, and I knew he meant it, "I love you, Dad. You're strong. You'll do as well as anybody could." As best I recall, he didn't say he knew I'd be fine. I'm glad he didn't, because he couldn't know that and I needed something more helpful than denial. When we hugged good-bye at the airport, we both held on a little longer than usual.

Neither Patricia nor I sleeps well on airplanes, so by the time we got back home about 8:00 A.M., we were totally spent. We knew we had to get at least two or three hours of sleep before going to work and fell into bed. Wordlessly, we clung to each other. Desperately and rather quickly, but with absolute communication, we made love as if it might be for the last time. Then we cried a little, unplugged the phone, and slept.

CHAPTER 3

DARKNESS

The afternoon was hard. I had my lecture ready, but I felt I was walking underwater. When I got back to the office after class, I talked for a bit with Rita, our departmental coordinator and a good friend as well. She had known about the biopsy and asked if I had heard anything. I gave her the bare-bones report, which was still all I had, and told her what Dr. Carlton had recommended. As one who has faced her share of problems with a strong coping spirit, she showed both concern and a matter-of-fact recognition that I now had to decide what to do. Before long, Steve and Chad also showed up and they, too, asked about the biopsy results. At hearing Carlton's recommendation, Steve observed that oncological surgeons he knew could make a good argument for snipping the offending tissue out. Chad, on the other hand, had read that, because prostate cancer tends to progress slowly, some doctors feel it is best not to do anything until a tumor proves to be truly dangerous. I told them I did not know what I was going to do, but asked them not to mention my situation to anyone for a few days, until I had a chance to sort things out. I wasn't trying to keep my condition a secret, but I wanted to avoid unnecessary sources of static while I was trying to get a clear signal.

That evening, I called our oldest son, Rex, who lives in Houston, and our daughter, Dale, who lives in Baton Rouge, where her husband Rupert works for Shell. I remembered my reaction at hearing my father tell me he had a fatal disease and even though I assured them there was little chance of my dying anytime soon and, indeed, that the chances of full recovery were excellent, I could imagine something of what they felt. Parents, in the orthodox version of life, have always been there, and life without them is difficult to imagine. Many young children acknowledge hoping they will die before their parents do, because they cannot bear the thought of being orphaned. Of course, as we get older and our dependence on parents decreases, we accept the sequential nature of generations and understand that they will eventually die, and that we will be able to handle it. Still, it can be a shock to contemplate having one's own generation move to the head of the line. Like Jeff, both Rex and Dale told me they loved me and urged me to do whatever it might take to get the best possible treatment. Both also said they would come see me soon.

Over the next two days, Thursday and Friday,

my spirits darkened. I figured I needed to tell Jim
Pomerantz, my dean, since whatever course of
treatment I chose, particularly if it was surgery,
would likely make it difficult for me to meet all
my responsibilities. He was immediately sympa-
thetic, assuring me that I should give my attention
to taking care of myself, and not worry about my
duties at Rice. He also told me that his brother-in-
law is a urologist and that he would ask him for
his counsel.

Thursday afternoon, I broke the news to another colleague, Elizabeth. Chad came in while we
were talking. Elizabeth asked just how big the
prostate gland is. With the assurance of men who
had one, we answered in concert, "About the size
of a walnut," and went on to fill her in on our previous conversations. We discussed our mutual
reluctance to rush to surgery unless it was
absolutely unavoidable, and I moved closer to
insisting to Dr. Carlton that I wanted radiation
therapy, even given the poorer odds of success.

Early Thursday morning, I had left a message at
David Bybee's office, asking that he call back
when he had a chance. When he returned my call
about 4:00, he was not surprised to hear my news.
"When I saw your message, I figured that was the
result," he said. I told him what Dr. Carlton had
recommended, which did not surprise him. Both
the estimated cure rates for surgery and radiation

and the recommendation of surgery, he said, were "the party line at Baylor." That was not a criticism. Though he acknowledged that "the last word has not been written," he felt these figures were the best available at present and said he leaned toward surgery in younger, healthy men.

I asked Dr. Bybee if Dr. Carlton would consider it a breach of protocol for me to get a second opinion at M. D. Anderson. He assured me it was perfectly proper and said he would set it up for me. He observed that Gene Carlton has given most of his professional life to the study of prostate cancer and does a great deal of continuing education on the subject for other physicians. Carlton, he said, uses a perineal approach for the surgery, getting at the prostate through an incision in the perineum, between the anus and the scrotum. This is less traumatic to the patient and results in less loss of blood, both of which contribute to a quicker recovery. It also seems to enable patients to regain continence more easily. In cases in which radiation is indicated, he said, Carlton favors the combination of radioactive implants followed by external beam radiation, believing that this makes it possible to reduce some of the complications that can accompany high doses of radiation. He added, however, that radiotherapists at both M. D. Anderson and Methodist Hospital feel they have learned how to control the external beam dosage sufficiently well to make the use of implants unnecessary.

Then, in his gentle but matter-of-fact way, David told me of his experience with other prostate cancer patients. It was not heartening. All those who had chosen surgery had been incontinent for a while, some for as long as two years. The best recovery he had seen had been in an athletic 62-year-old who had returned to work in three weeks and was fully continent in three months. David knew that Carlton and his colleagues claimed to preserve sexual function in at least half their cases, but that had not been his experience. In fact, only one patient had recovered sufficient potency for intercourse, and that was with "reduced tumescence." Others had resorted to injections in the penis—"to prime the pump"— and to inflatable penile implants.

The results for radiation were no more reassuring. Incontinence was not usually much of a threat, but the treatment often led to impotence in a fairly short time. Most of his patients had experienced some problems with diarrhea and proctitis (inflammation of the rectum), particularly in the latter phase of the treatment. At one time in the remote past, a patient's rectum had been burned so badly by the radiation that he had required a diverting colostomy. In another case, the radiation had caused elephantisis of the scrotum, causing it to swell up to the size of a basketball. "It was quite painful," he noted, an observation that did not surprise me. I asked how long that condition had lasted. "It didn't go down. And they couldn't operate on it. He was like that the rest of his life. It was awkward." David Bybee has no talent for hyperbole.

I sensed that Dr. Bybee felt bad about giving me such dreadful news, but I appreciated his candor. I told him that and I also told him I was grateful to him for insisting I have the biopsy. In keeping with his character, he responded softly, "I'm sorry I didn't think of it two years earlier."

Thursday evening, I attended a meeting at which I learned that the major part of a sizable investment I had made several years earlier was about to go down the tubes. While definitely not good news, it was not the worst I had received that week, and I found it hard to get too worked up about it. After the meeting, I sat in a car and shared my news with Mary Lee, a fellow investor and dear friend. I knew well that she and her husband Sidney loved Patricia and me, but I was pleased to have her reaffirm that fact, and to know that they would be standing with us through whatever we had to face.

Late that evening, I decided to take advantage of one of the great benefits of being a university professor and tapped into the treasure-trove of

information available via my computer. I knew
Rice was hooked into the Texas Medical Center,
but I didn't know much beyond that, so I was
mainly on a fishing expedition. Before long, I had
followed the Internet trail to something called
PDQ, for Physician's Data Query. This service
provides physicians with a synthesis of continually updated material, mostly from medical journals, on a wide range of medical topics. I saw
immediately that this was an informational gold
mine. When I burrowed my way to "cancer," and
then to "prostate cancer," I found dozens of pages
of densely packed material, too much to try to
digest right then, but too intensely relevant to
leave without dipping in here and there. An hour
or so later, I knew that prostate cancer can be sorted into stages A, B, C, and D, and that, as in real
life, an A is much better than a D. I read the percentages on five- and ten- and fifteen-year survival rates. And then, I found the first truly good
news I had heard in a while. In 1982, a Dr. Patrick
Walsh at Johns Hopkins had developed a "nerve-
sparing" surgical technique that greatly reduced
the incidence of both incontinence and impotence,
especially in men under sixty. I was sleepy and
had to quit, but I knew I wanted to learn more
about Dr. Walsh—PDQ. I told the computer I
would like a printed copy of this information, and
it told me I could pick it up the next day at the

computer center.

The next morning, Sidney called to express his concern and to tell me about Franz, a colleague and mutual friend who had gone through radiation treatment at Baylor and had declared it a complete success. I had neither known of this nor been able to pinpoint any time when Franz had been out of commission, a circumstance I regarded as a vote in favor of radiation therapy. I called Franz right away and he confirmed what Sidney had said. Four years earlier, a urologist had implanted a radioactive "seed" in his prostate. After a few days in the hospital—not because he needed the time to recover, but to protect others while the seed was still emitting high levels of radiation—he received brief daily doses of external radiation for several weeks. It had been easy, his PSA had dropped well into the normal range and he seemed to be doing fine. I told him of Dr. Carlton's recommendation that I have the surgery and of the respective odds he had assigned to surgery and radiation. I observed that surviving was quite important to me, but that the quality of life was also important.

"You're damn tootin'!" he shot back.

Without prying, but to make sure he knew exactly what I was talking about, I said that I was worried that the surgery might destroy sexual function.

"You're damn tootin'!" he repeated. He knew exactly what I was talking about. Another vote for radiation, I thought.

Sidney had also reminded me that another of our colleagues, Sam, had been diagnosed with prostate cancer a few months earlier. I knew Sam had some kind of cancer, but he was on sabbatical in Washington, and I had not had a good opportunity to talk with him. I sent him an e-mail message immediately and soon received a brief but informative reply. He was on his way to a conference and didn't have time to go into detail, but he would be in touch the following week to explain why, after months of research and uncertainty, he had decided to have the surgery.

Within an hour, Jim Pomerantz dropped by my office to report that his brother-in-law had said that surgery was clearly the route I should take and, further, that "no responsible urologist in the country would give you any different advice." He had also volunteered that Gene Carlton and his colleague, Peter Scardino, current head of the Department of Urology of Baylor, were widely regarded as two of the best in the world.

This was not getting easier.

I met my class again Friday afternoon. This was the hardest specific task I had. Regardless of one's grasp of the subject, some element of performance is involved in teaching a class of 120 students effectively. It was difficult to perform. As I stood waiting for the elevator to take me downstairs, I would have paid a substantial sum to have the next hour pass in a flash, without my having to go through it. When I reached the classroom, the water level still seemed to be up near the ceiling. I got through it, because I work from rather full lecture notes and I had done most of the preparation before we left for California, but if teaching were as hard as that every day, I would look for another job.

Before the day was over, I told my little story to my two remaining sociology colleagues, Angela and Chandler, and to Julie, an anthropologist whose office is just down the hall and who happened to ask me how everything was going. Angela and Julie hugged me, which did not surprise me. So did Chandler, which did. I met Chandler the first day I came to Rice, in 1968, and except when one of us was on sabbatical or vacation, I have seen him most days since then. We know what the other thinks on most issues, and the correlation between our views, though not perfect, is statistically significant. More remarkably, I cannot recall that either of us has ever directed an unpleasant word toward the other. So I was not surprised to see that Chandler was stunned to see that his colleague of longest standing had cancer. Though we understood that one of us would one day be the first to fall victim to some dread malady or accident, it probably never occurred to Chandler that I might be the one. It had certainly never occurred to me. We talked about the prospects and the leading options until there was not much else to say. As I got up to leave, he came around from behind his desk, gave me a big bear hug, and said, "Buddy, I don't know what to say, but I'll do whatever I can. You know that." He'd never called me "Buddy" before, either.

On Friday evening, I called my sister, Helen, who lives in Baltimore. I had not left her off the list of people who needed to be contacted, but she is hard to reach except on Friday nights and Sundays. She teaches school full time during the day, then attends nursing school almost every evening and Saturday. She is a great teacher and she will be a great nurse. She is tougher than I am by several degrees. Certainly she has dealt with a greater range of challenges. In addition to her own five children, three acquired when she married a widower shortly after graduating from college, she and her husband have been foster parents for more than 70 children, nearly all of whom came to them from the juvenile courts, where Dick was a judge and she a key administrator. After leaving the juvenile system, she served for several years as an adult probation officer. She has had serious health problems, as has her family. My life has gone more smoothly and, although I don't think she holds that against me, she has noted from time to time that I seem to have a golden horseshoe embedded in the lower part of my body. Helen is a care giver of monumental capacity, and her friends love her for it, but she is not particularly generous with unnecessary sympathy. When she answered the phone, I told her, after introductory exchanges, that my horseshoe had broken.

"What's wrong?" she asked.

"I have cancer."

"What kind?"

"Prostate."

"Aw, that's not so bad. If you have to have cancer, that's the one to get."

I had come to expect having my friends and relatives react with shock and concern for my welfare, and to express the dismay they felt at conceiving of a world without me. But Helen, exercising one of her chief gifts, ministered to my head rather than to my heart. She was sorry, of course, but she knew I had work to do and she was ready to help. She told me she would talk to some doctors and nurses the next day, and would go to the medical library and copy some articles for me. She ventured that my horseshoe was only bent, not broken, and that I could count on recovering.

And then she told me what I had never doubted—
that she, like my more sentimental friends, also
loved me.

CHAPTER 4

LIGHT

Patricia, who oversees international students and study abroad programs at Rice, was scheduled to attend a conference in Mexico City over the weekend. She was extremely reluctant to leave me at this point, but had been newly elected to an office and was scheduled to give a presentation. She also felt an obligation to a colleague who taken the lead role in organizing the conference. I urged her to go, feeling confident I was in little danger of dropping into serious depression in her absence. Not long after she left for the airport on Saturday morning, I climbed on my bicycle and headed for the main library in the Texas Medical Center. As soon as I learned how to navigate the search computer and the *Index Medicus*, a major reference work similar to the *Readers Guide*, I drew up a three-page list of articles and books and dived into a sea of medical lore. I didn't come up for air or food or drink other than water for nine hours, and part of that time was spent photocopying several inches of material that would occupy me for the rest of the weekend.

One of the reasons I became a sociologist is that,

since there is a sociology of virtually everything, one has wide latitude as to what constitutes a proper object of study. That makes it easy to recover the curiosity and excitement that led me, at age sixteen, to decide I wanted to be a college professor, even though I had little idea as to what it was I might want to profess. By noon, I was totally engrossed in trying to unravel the riddles of prostate cancer, sometimes almost to the point of forgetting just why I had developed such a keen interest in the subject. For four days, I had worried about incontinence and impotence and, of course, death. Now I realized I had another first-rate reason for wanting to whip this intruder in my life: I want to keep on looking stuff up and trying to make sense of it for as long as I can.

I began with overview articles that filled in some of the gaps in my prostate lore. I learned that the "gland" is composed not only of tiny, glandular structures, but also of muscle and connective tissue known as stroma. The outer surface, called the prostatic capsule, is muscle. Though nothing actually separates them, it is common to speak of "zones" or "lobes" within the prostate: a central zone surrounding the urethra, a peripheral zone surrounding that, and a small transitional zone within the central lobe, next to the urethral sphincter. In a young boy, the prostate is about the size of a bean. It grows slowly until puberty, then rapidly until a man reaches his twenties. At mature size, it weighs about 20 grams and is, as noted, "about the size of a walnut." Then it stops growing—for awhile. By the time men reach their mid-forties, it starts to grow again and, in most cases, continues to grow until death. A small percentage of men escape this aggravation. Since some of these men have less facial and body hair and also do not become bald, their good fortune on this score is probably related to a low level of androgens—male hormones. Not all men would trade conditions.

In most cases, the gland's size increases by only about 50 percent. This may or may not cause problems. The key is the pattern of growth. Recall that the urethra runs right through the middle of the gland, like a straw. If the new growth is outward and does not pinch the straw, a man may experience few noticeable symptoms, even when the growth is larger than normal. If the growth is inward, pinching the straw, a little bit can go a long way, producing the familiar symptoms of BPH: frequent urination, nocturia (nighttime urination), difficulty in starting the stream, a meager stream, a dribbling stop, uncomfortable urgency, and an inability to empty the bladder completely, which can lead to infection, though this is rare. About half of men over 50 experience some of the symptoms of BPH. By age 70, the rate rises to around 75 percent, and continues to rise as men get older. It is a notable inconvenience, and is estimated to account for approximately 1.7 million doctor visits and 400,000 operations annually.[1] As one writer put it, this little gland "causes more misery for men than just about any other structure in the body."[2]

Urologists recommend that men suffering from BPH take such sensible measures as minimizing liquid intake in the evening, cutting down on caffeine and alcohol, and trying to be sure they empty their bladders each time they urinate. Drugs such as Hytrin and Proscar may help. Antihistamines, decongestants, and some tranquilizers and antidepressants can aggravate the condition. Since prostate growth, normal and abnormal, is dependent upon testosterone, hormonal treatments that inhibit the production of testosterone can help. So, of course, can castration. For the present, however, the "gold standard" for treating BPH is still the Roto-Rooter, known more formally as a transurethral resection of the prostate, or TURP.

As one might guess from its "Roto-Rooter" nickname, a TURP is performed by inserting a resectoscope through the penis and urethra to the inside of the prostate. This remarkable instrument includes a light, a cutting instrument (usually a knife or electrical current, though lasers have recently been used), electrical current to cauterize blood vessels, and irrigating tubes to flush resected tissue back out through the penis. Doesn't seem like it would all fit, does it? Working from the inside outward, the surgeon removes BPH tissue, which can be distinguished from normal tissue, a little bit at a time until the patient is left with only his original-equipment gland. The inch or so of urethra running through the prostate is destroyed, but it grows back.

Hundreds of thousands of TURPS are performed in America every year, at an estimated total cost of over $3 billion (at $6,000–8,000 per case), most of it paid by Medicare, since patients tend to be older. Even so, it is not like having one's appendix removed. Much can go wrong, and between .3 and 1.0 percent (depending on whose data one accepts) of TURP patients die as a direct or indirect result of the operation. Most of these deaths occur outside major hospitals, underscoring the observation of a physician/researcher who cautioned that "[TURP] must be learned with painstaking care; it is an operation for the dedicated professional with no place for the enthusiastic amateur."[3]

Fascinating as I found it, since I was also a BPH victim, I began to skip over this material and concentrate on cancer. Not only was this scarier, but I discovered much less agreement among physicians as to what should be done.

In any kind of carcinoma, cancer cells multiply in an out-of-control manner, overcoming and destroying adjoining healthy cells. A cancer can be primary or secondary; that is, it can originate at the site or spread from another site. Prostate cancer is almost always primary, but often metastasizes (spreads) through the lymph nodes to other parts of the body, particularly the bones. If it spreads widely, it may be controlled for a time, but it cannot be cured by current therapy. Because it is typically a slow-growing cancer that tends to afflict older men, many of its victims die from other causes before it can run its course or even cause serious symptoms, giving rise to the common observation that "more men die with prostate cancer than of it."

The median age of prostate cancer victims in the U.S. is being revised downward rather rapidly. The conventional figure has been 72. Several authorities gave 67 as a more accurate mid-point, and at least one asserted that it might be as low as 62. To a considerable extent, this lowering of the median age reflects more aggressive screening by physicians, particularly since the advent of the PSA test. Because many men have failed to be tested routinely for prostate cancer, and because the disease typically manifests few or no symp-

toms until it is well developed, a multitude of
cases that are now caught early would previously
have gone undetected until the men were several
years older. Similarly, part of the rising incidence
of the disease—an estimated 165,000 cases were
newly diagnosed in 1993, the estimate for 1994 is
200,000 cases as compared to less than 100,000 in
1990—is surely attributable to the fact that more
men are living longer because of a healthier
lifestyle and more advanced medicine. A generation or two earlier, many men died of heart disease or lung cancer before they were old enough
to get prostate cancer. Still, something else may
also be at work. Approximately 35,000 American
men died of prostate cancer in 1993, and the
American Cancer Society expects 38,000 to suc-
cumb to the disease in 1994, compared to only
24,000 in 1988. An increase of almost fifty percent
in five years gives credence to the view that we
are experiencing an epidemic of this disease. The
four-percent annual rate of increase since 1980 is
faster than that for any other cancer except skin
cancer, and, given the location of the prostate, it
seems unlikely that depletion of the ozone layer is
much of a factor.

It is surely true that the PSA test will call attention to many cancers that might pose little risk to
their hosts. Data collected from autopsies indicate
that the prostates of as many as one-third of men

over 50 show microscopic evidence of cancer, yet even the strongest advocates of aggressive treatment of the disease admit that most of these men could have waited years before their cancer posed any real danger, if it ever did. The conventional wisdom at present is that approximately one in nine American men will incur a significant form of the disease in their lifetimes, and that perhaps as many as eighty percent of those will be over sixty-five. (I was pleasantly struck by the fact that urological journals routinely refer to anyone under sixty-five as young. Two days later, I read an article in *Fortune* magazine, in which the author, Tom Alexander, made the same observation. Since he was sixty-two and therefore rapidly approaching the end of his days as a youth, I resolved not to resent his beating me to the line.)[4]

For reasons not well understood, the prevalence of prostate cancer varies widely from place to place, and from population to population within the same region, though environment does seem to play an important role. This generalization, however, requires an important qualification. Evidence from autopsies—the same kind of data that indicate one-third of American men in their fifties have at least traces of the disease—reveals a remarkable similarity in the prevalence of detectable cancer cells (histologic disease) in the prostates of men from every region and every ethnic group studied. One could reasonably expect that rates of "clinically evident disease" (disease a physician could diagnose) and "disease-specific mortality" (deaths actually traceable to prostate cancer) would also be similar across regions and groups. Since the opposite is true, it seems reasonable to believe that environmental factors must play a key role in allowing or encouraging the microscopic cancer cells to develop to threatening dimensions.[5]

The highest rates are in Scandinavia and North America; the lowest in Asia and Eastern Europe, with England, Southern Europe, and South America in between. The differences can be astonishing. Swedish men, for example, are 220 times more likely to suffer from prostate cancer than are Hondurans, and residents of Alameda County, California, have a rate 125 times that of Shanghai. In Israel, rates among Jews vary with their country of origin.[6] One of the highest rates in the world belongs to African-Americans—77 cases per 100,000 black males (of all ages). In sharp contrast, Nigerian and Senagalese blacks have rates of only 10 and 4.3 per 100,000 respectively. When Nigerians and Senegalese move to the United States, however, their rates of prostate cancer rise approximately tenfold. Similarly, though native Japanese men have an incidence rate of only 4 per 100,000, the rate for Japanese living on the U.S. mainland ranges between 12 and 20 per 100,000, and the rate for those living in Hawaii is 36 per 100,000. A comparable pattern occurs among Chinese men, with minuscule rates in Shanghai, higher rates in Hong Kong and Singapore, and much higher rates in the U.S.

Some of the differences in rates is quite likely traceable to differences in diagnostic practices and access to good treatment. For example, the overall incidence rate for America is 42 per 100,000, while the rate for Britain is only 19 per 100,000. The rates of death from prostate cancer, however, are much closer—15 per 100,000 for the U.S. and 12 per 100,000 for Britain. More aggressive screening for prostate cancer turns up more cases in the U.S., but the proportion of cases serious enough to cause death are similar. Access to treatment almost surely explains the fact that American blacks are significantly more likely than American whites to die from prostate cancer. Because, for economic and other reasons, they are less likely to seek treatment until serious symptoms present themselves, blacks may not discover they have prostate cancer until it is too far advanced to cure.[7]

Since progressively higher rates can be seen in successive generations of immigrant families, environment must be a critical factor, with a

"Western" diet high in red meat and dairy products an especially likely contributor. A high-fat diet may either raise the testosterone level or reduce the prostate's resistance to the cancer-stimulating testosterone. In any case, and for other health-related reasons as well, men are well advised to cut down on fats and increase their intake of grains, fruits, and green and yellow vegetables.[8] Regular exercise and weight control may also help, both in preventing cancer and in giving those who develop it a better chance of survival.

Diet is not the only plausible culprit. Within the United States, certain occupations correlate with higher rates of prostate cancer. Painters, printers, rubber workers, electroplaters, battery makers, drug and chemical workers, and farmers all have higher than average rates. They are also all exposed to a variety of chemicals and toxins. Less easy to explain is the higher-than-average incidence of the disease among bookkeepers, shipping clerks, and people in personnel services. Perhaps sitting on one's prostate all day long is counterproductive.[9]

Numerous other possible associations have been explored, with mixed results. Some studies have indicated that men who have had a vasectomy run a markedly higher risk—in one study, 66 percent higher—of getting prostate cancer than men who have not, but more recent data cast serious doubt on this association.[10] Heredity definitely appears to play a role. A man whose father had prostate cancer, particularly if he had it before he was 65, is more than twice as likely to develop the disease than the average man. If more than one relative has had it, the risk is even higher.[11] I am sorry that is the case, but at least I know my two sons will heed Senator Robert Dole's eloquent admonition to "be on the lookout for this stuff."[12] Smokers do not seem to have an increased risk of prostate cancer, perhaps because a substantial proportion of them die of heart disease or lung cancer before prostate cancer has a chance to develop.

Early sexual activity, venereal disease, extensive extra-marital activity, and frequent visits to prostitutes have also been implicated, but the studies are poor and the data inconsistent. Even if such correlations were consistently reported, the explanation for all of them might be, to put it plainly, testosterone poisoning. Once again, the data are inconsistent, with some studies showing a positive correlation between high testosterone levels and prostate cancer but with others failing to confirm it. Still, while the exact role of androgens (male hormones, including testosterone), is uncertain, it is a fact that eunuchs don't get prostate cancer.[13] I wouldn't care to defend any of the activities mentioned in the above list, and, as a part-time criminologist, I firmly believe that testosterone is implicated in a lion's share of crime and violence. Still, I was not entirely chagrined to read these studies.

Years ago, I asked the bass singer of the famed Statesmen gospel quartet why it is that women always seem to be attracted to the bass singers in such groups. He hemmed and hawed a bit, then allowed that, "I think they kind of understand that, well, you just can't sing bass and be a sissy, if you know what I mean." I have never thought of myself as a middle-aged stud, and I have grown accustomed to being invisible to most women whom I did not know. Still, I rather enjoyed being a balding grandfather sufficiently virile to please a lovely and loving wife, and I recognized that I preferred to have a disease related to the presence of testosterone rather than to its absence. Like singing bass, prostate cancer is not for sissies.

Prostatic tumors are commonly described as slow-growing, but experts differ in their opinions of just how slow, and whether some grow much faster than others.

One of the leading figures in the field, Dr. Thomas Stamey of Stanford University School of Medicine, contends that, once true cancer cells have developed, they will continue to grow and multiply at a relatively uniform, though slow, rate. He estimates that about ten years is required for a microscopic carcinoma to grow into a tumor with a volume of one cubic centimeter. If this were true, it would be fairly simple to obtain a rough calculation of how long a man with a tiny tumor could wait until deciding to do something about it. Stamey's view, however, is a minority opinion. Since the incidence of microscopic disease is quite similar throughout the world, Stamey's hypothesis would predict similar rates of full-blown cancer in all groups. We know that is not the case. It seems to follow, then, either that some cancer cells are intrinsically more aggressive than others or that some factors, whether genetic or environmental or both, stimulate more rapid malignant growth.[14]

The inability to predict how a given malignancy is going to behave constitutes a major dilemma for both physicians and patients. Because the current major forms of treatment—surgery, radiation, and hormonal therapy—all pose a significant threat to sexual function and can have other negative results, including death, many experts recommend a course of "expectant management" or "watchful waiting." These synonymous terms refer to an approach in which a patient diagnosed with prostate cancer may choose to do nothing other than make regular visits to his urologist, who will keep his finger on the situation. If the tumor grows, then action may need to be taken. If

it doesn't, the patient can avoid the negative
effects of treatment for several years, and perhaps
for the rest of his life. The gamble is that one will
wait too long, and that by the time physician and
patient decide more aggressive action is required,
it will be too late. The cancer will have spread
outside the gland and become incurable.
Physicians advocating an aggressive approach to
the disease contend that every prostate cancer is at
some point confined to the gland. If it can be
detected while it is still confined, it can probably
be cured, giving the man a good chance to live a
normal life span. If it has spread to the lymph
nodes in the pelvic region, but not beyond, at the
time of detection, the patient has a 50 to 60 percent chance of living 10 years. If it spreads to the
bones or other organs, such as the lungs or liver,
the chances of surviving longer than 5 years drop
to 30 percent. More conservative physicians do
not necessarily disagree with this, but feel there is
no reason to rush to treatment until the signs
clearly warrant it. The most frequently quoted
expression of this dilemma has been formulated
by one of the giants of urological research,
Memorial Sloan-Kettering's Willet F. Whitmore,
Jr., who notes that urologists face the difficult
question, "Is cure necessary in those in whom it
may be possible, and is cure possible in those in
whom it is necessary?"[15]

Despite the fact that both Drs. Bybee and Carlton had recommended surgery, I was determined to explore radiation and "watchful waiting" a bit further before surrendering to the knife. I soon discovered that European doctors are far more likely than their American counterparts to take a conservative approach to prostate cancer. In part, this reflects economic necessity. As more and more men live long enough to become vulnerable to the disease, extensive resort to either surgery or radiation could place an enormous burden on tax-supported national health programs. Since most victims of the disease are older men who might well die of other causes before the cancer gets them, the argument goes, aggressive treatment may not lengthen their lives and may even decrease the quality of their lives in the years they do have left. In addition, many European physicians appear to think that Americans feel obliged to do *something* even if doing *nothing* might produce an equally satisfactory, if not better, result. Deep down, I suspected I did not have the temperament for watchful waiting. If that's because I'm an American, so be it. But my first four days with cancer had been hard ones, and I seriously doubted I would be content to play the blithe host to a potentially dangerous tumor for very long. Still, I needed to find out just how bad my situation was. That led me to explore the grading and staging of prostate cancer.

My dean's urologist brother-in-law had asked him if I knew what my Gleason score was. I had never heard the term, so I was on the lookout for it. Prostate cancers are graded according to how well "differentiated" they are. The better the differentiation, the better the prognosis; other things being equal, a tumor that resembles a BB, or even a small marble, is less dangerous than one that looks like a piece of squashed goat cheese. As they grow and spread, cancers usually become poorly differentiated—looking more like a fungus or a piece of runny cheese than a BB. To facilitate choice of appropriate treatment, several grading systems have been developed. The most widely used was developed by Dr. Donald F. Gleason in 1966. Gleason identified five grades of tumor.

Grade 1 tumors are small and quite well differentiated, like BBs. Though they can be distinguished from normal prostate tissue, they closely resemble normal glands. They do not deform the small glands within the prostate.

Grade 2 tumors are also well-defined, but not so sharply as Grade 1. They are somewhat larger and vary more in size and shape than do normal glands.

Grade 3 tumors vary even more widely in size and shape and are moderately differentiated, moving out into the stroma of the prostate like the edges of a growing fungus.

Grade 4 tumors consist of large, densely packed malignant cells that are spread throughout the stroma of the prostate, noticeably deforming the glandular structure.

Grade 5 tumors are quite undifferentiated, spreading throughout the prostate and destroying most or all of the glandular structure.

The final Gleason score—not the *grade*, but the *score*—is obtained by adding the grade of the two most common patterns found in the biopsied tissue. If only one grade is identified, its number is doubled to obtain the Gleason score. Possible scores range between 2 (a doubled 1) and 10 (a doubled 5). Cancers scored in the 2 to 4 range are well-differentiated, those in the 5 to 7 range are moderately differentiated, and those scored 8 to 10 are considered poorly differentiated. These clusters of scores correlate well, though not perfectly, with metastasis, elevated PSA and serum enzymatic acid phosphatase levels, and with chances of survival. The higher the score, the worse the prognosis.[16]

A key advantage of the Gleason system is that pathologists do not need sophisticated equipment to employ it. Biopsied tissue is examined visually through a standard laboratory microscope. A major disadvantage of the system is the substantial degree of subjectivity involved in assigning a grade. Several tests have demonstrated that experienced pathologists can disagree over the proper grade to assign a given tumor. In one extensive study, pathologists tutored by Gleason himself rendered identical verdicts on only 38 percent of a large number of cases. When the same pathologists, including Gleason, reviewed the same slides for a second time, they agreed with their first assessment in only about 80 percent of the cases. Even so, the final score differed by more than one point on only 18 percent of the cases.[17] Without benefit of a microscope or tissue sample, I decided that my tumor, since it had not been detected by DRE or ultrasound, could not possibly have a Gleason grade worse than 3. A grade of 1 or 2 seemed far more likely.

Closely correlated with a tumor's grade is its stage. Once again, a variety of staging systems exist, but two predominate over all others. The first is known variously as the Whitmore-Jewett, or ABCD, system. Whitmore delineated four stages of prostatic carcinoma, which he labeled ABCD. Hugh J. Jewett elaborated on this scheme by subdividing the stages into A1 and A2, B1 and B2, etc. This system, with further refinements, has long been the one favored by most American urologists. The other classification device, known as the TNM system—the letters stand for Tumor, Node, and Metastasis—is favored in Europe. It is coming into wide use in the U.S., not only because of its utility, but also to facilitate comparative research. In both systems, stages are reported as either clinical or pathological. Clinical staging is based on DRE, TRUS, biopsied tissue, and such tests of metastasis as bone scans and MRIs (magnetic resonance imaging). It is done in an effort to determine how extensive a cancer is and, therefore, what kinds of treatment are appropriate. Pathological staging is based on more extensive examination of tissue after the prostate is removed surgically, or as part of an autopsy. Clinical staging is less precise than pathological staging, and it is fairly common for the latter to reveal that the carcinoma was worse than the clinical staging had estimated.

I made little effort to understand the European system during this early encounter with it, and I did not get a firm hold on the ABCD system for several days, but this is a good place to sketch the main features of each system. A comparative table in the appendix may also be useful to some readers.

Stage A tumors are those detected not by DRE or TRUS, but by pathological examination of tissue specimens obtained, for example, during a Roto-Rooter operation or extracted because of suspicion raised by a high PSA reading. **A1** tumors are well-differentiated and occupy less than 5 percent of the tissue specimen. **A2** tumors occupy more than 5 percent of the tissue or are moderately or poorly differentiated. Most Stage A cancers are curable. Many physicians consider Stage A1 tumors to be perfect prospects for watchful waiting. Others consider them ideal candidates for aggressive therapy, since the likelihood of cure is excellent. Before the PSA test came into wide use, physicians were unlikely to discover Stage A tumors, for the simple reason that, in the absence of symptoms or any abnormal formation a doctor could feel during a DRE, there was little reason to call for a biopsy. Predictably, a significant amount of the rising incidence of prostate cancer comprises Stage A tumors discovered in biopsies ordered after abnormal PSA readings.

Stage B prostatic cancer can be detected by a digital exam. If there is a single nodule, no larger than two centimeters at its greatest dimension and confined to one lobe of the prostate, the cancer is regarded as a **B1**. A well-differentiated B1 tumor may offer better prospects for cure than a less well-differentiated A2 tumor. If the tumor is larger than 2 centimeters or if there is more than one tumor, but the cancer has apparently not penetrated the prostatic capsule, it is classified as **B2**. A **B3** tumor involves both the central and peripheral lobes. Long-term data have indicated that metastasis to the lymph nodes will have occurred in almost 20 percent of B1 tumors and approximately one-third of B2 and B3 tumors by the time they are discovered. Increasingly, these figures are being seen as too pessimistic. As more men become aware of the need for prostatic examinations, more Stage B tumors are being caught before they escape from the capsule, with the result that recent data reflect metastasis in about 5 percent of B1 tumors and 10 to 15 percent of B2 and B3 tumors. Still, because most Stage B tumors produce no symptoms, men who fail to get regular physical exams or who refuse to allow their doctors to perform a DRE may not discover they have prostate cancer until it has become incurable. Most Stage B cancers, however, are potentially curable.

By the time they reach **Stage C**, prostatic tumors are decidedly more dangerous. They are larger and extend beyond the prostatic capsule, but show no evidence of metastasis and are therefore still potentially curable. **C1** tumors are smaller than 6 centimeters in diameter; **C2** tumors are larger. They may or may not produce symptoms, depending mainly on whether the growth impinges on the urethra. Though a Stage C cancer may have extended into the walls of the capsule, the seminal vesicles, and the base of the bladder, it has—by definition—not metastasized to the lymph nodes, the bones, or other organs. In fact, however, about half of all prostate cancers initially classified as Stage C will have spread, requiring reclassification into **Stage D**. When the cancerous growth has spread to the lymph nodes but not beyond, it is labeled a **D1**. When metastasis has occurred beyond the nodes, it is classified as **D2** and is considered incurable, though palliative treatment can keep a patient alive for a number of years. Stage C cancers can be treated by surgery, radiation, or hormone therapy.

Until the advent of the PSA test, more than 40 percent of all prostate cancers had already reached Stage D by the time they were first diagnosed. In a high proportion of these cases, men have come to their doctors not because of urinary difficulties, but because of bone pain (usually in the spine, but sometimes in the pelvis, hips, or upper legs), a sign the disease has reached a late point in its natural history. Most, but not all, physicians believe that neither radiation nor surgery are likely to prove effective with a Stage D tumor. Because almost all prostate cancers are dependent on testosterone for continued growth, reduction or elimination of testosterone production will often check a Stage D cancer and extend a patient's life by several years. The two most common means of checking production are hormone therapy and castration, known in the trade as orchiectomy or, occasionally, orchidectomy.[18]

The TNM system provides labels that are more precise than those of the ABCD scheme, since each variable—Tumor, Node, and Metastasis—is assigned a stage, producing a summary designation that yields considerable information. The T(umor) rankings are similar to those in the Whitmore-Jewett system. The N(ode) rankings indicate whether or not a cancer has spread to the lymph nodes and, if so, how extensively. The M(etastasis) ranking indicates the degree of metastasis, if any. A 1992 revision of the system, adopted by both the International Union Against Cancer and the American Joint Committee on Cancer, recognizes the following tumor stages.

Tumor Status

T-Zero: No evidence of primary tumor

T1: Tumors not detectable by DRE or TRUS (as Stage A tumors). These can be of three types:

   T1a: Tumor an incidental finding in 5 percent or less of tissue removed in treatment of BPH.

   T1b: Tumor an incidental finding in more than 5 percent of tissue removed in treatment of BPH

   T1c: Tumor identified by needle biopsy, usually taken because of elevated serum PSA.

T2: Tumor is detectable by DRE or TRUS, but is confined within the prostate (as Stage B tumors). Again, there are three sub-types:

T2a: Tumor involves half of one lobe or less.

T2b: Tumor involves more than half of one lobe, but not both lobes.

T2c: Tumor involves both lobes.

T3: Tumor extends through the prostate capsule (as in Stage C).

T3a: Extension through only one side of the capsule.

T3b: Extension through both sides.

T3c: Extension into the seminal vesicles.

T4: Tumor invades adjacent structures other than the seminal vesicles (as in Stages C and D)

T4a: Extension to bladder neck and/or external sphincter and/or rectum.

T4b: Tumor invades surrounding muscles and/or is fixed to the pelvic wall.

Nodal status is classified as follows:

NX and N-zero: Lymph nodes not assessed (X) or not involved (zero).

N1:ᐟ Cancer extends to one node, in the immediate region of the prostate.

N2:   Multiple nodes involved.

N3:   Involvement of fixed nodal mass not attached to the tumor.

N4:   Cancer extends to nodes in other regions of the body.

Metastasic status

MX and M-zero: Metastasis not assessed (X) or not present (zero)

M1a: Biochemical evidence of metastasis.

M1b: Single metastasis in single organ site (e.g., liver or lungs)

M1c: Multiple metastasis in single site.

M1d: Multiple metastatic sites.

When the three indicators are combined, they yield considerable information. For example, a prostate cancer labeled T1c-N0-M0 would be one discovered by needle biopsy, with neither nodal involvement nor evident metastasis. One labeled T3c-N2-M1c would indicate a patient has a tumor that extends into the seminal vesicles, beyond that into two or more lymph nodes, and shows evidence of multiple metastasis in a single organ. This greater precision makes it possible to conduct more meaningful research into the outcomes of various forms of therapy.[19]

A major reason for developing schemes to classify prostatic tumors is to provide physicians and patients with guidance as to the appropriate therapy. Surgical treatment would be useless on a cancer rated D or T4 with an N and M rating of 1 or greater, because it has already metastasized to other parts of the body. There is no point in subjecting a man to a major surgical procedure that would probably decrease the quality of his life while doing little or nothing to help his disease. At the other end of the spectrum, some A1/T1 tumors might be good candidates for "watchful waiting," particularly if the patient is elderly. Tumors of the middle range—palpable but still confined to the prostate, and perhaps even those that extend beyond the prostatic capsule but show no evidence of metastasis—call for harder choices. Some could undoubtedly be managed expectantly and left alone until they start to grow. Others, if not attacked aggressively, will kill their hosts. Informed medical opinion is sharply divided on the issue of treatment versus watchful waiting, with a substantial and perhaps increasing number of physicians adopting the watchful-waiting approach. Somewhat to my surprise, there is less disagreement on the question of surgery versus radiation.

In my long day's journey into light, I found nothing to contradict Dr. Carlton's recommendation of surgery as the appropriate treatment for

me. Over the short term—five years, perhaps
even as long as ten—survival figures for radiation
therapy approximate those for surgery. Beyond
that, the results of radiation therapy are simply
not as good as those obtained by surgery at the
hands of an expert. It now appears that, in
patients who live longer than ten years after irradiation, the cancer returns in at least 50 percent,
and perhaps as many as 80 percent, a far more
pessimistic estimate than the 70 percent success
rate Dr. Carlton had given me. Large-scale studies
of each method produce somewhat different overall figures, but surgery always comes out ahead
over longer periods. Most of the studies reported
in medical journals are conducted at research hospitals and do not include results obtained by less
expert physicians working in less prestigious and
less well-equipped settings, in which both surgery
and radiation are likely to yield poorer outcomes,
but there is no reason to think the relative differences between approaches would not persist.
Since mortality tables indicate that a man of 55
can expect to live another 20 to 22 years, surgery
clearly made sense in my case.

In a way, this was a relief. Over the years, I
have read various articles warning of the danger
of X-rays, so the prospect of absorbing 6,000-7,000
rads (roughly equivalent to 35,000 dental X-rays
or 1,000,000 chest X-rays) over a period of five or

six weeks discouraged me. I had considered irradiation a viable option only because I assumed it
offered a better chance of preserving sexual function. When I read that at least 50 percent of men
become impotent within a few months after radiation therapy for prostate cancer, and that some
studies report impotence rates in excess of 80 percent, I found it far less appealing. This information was now joined by journal references to a
substantial proportion—10 to 15 percent—of men
whom irradiation turns into "urological cripples"
with an urgent need to urinate every ten or fifteen
minutes. I knew these were unlikely outcomes,
and more recent data indicate that improved techniques have reduced their incidence to 2 to 3 percent, but they sounded awful.[20]

Why, then, would anyone opt for radiation
rather than surgery? Several good reasons exist.
The surgery—a radical prostatectomy—is a rough
one. The mortality rate for the surgery is 0.6
percent; at top-rated hospitals, however, only 0.1
percent of patients die from it, and few of these
deaths occur among men under 65.[21] For older
men with a shorter life expectancy or specific
health problems such as heart trouble, or even
less-than-robust general health, radiation is a
kinder, gentler option, with excellent short- and
middle-range results. In fact, most experienced
surgeons prefer not to perform a prostatectomy on

men with a life expectancy of less than ten years. Some place the cutoff point as low as 60 or 65, many use 70 as a rule of thumb, and many will make an exception in the case of a vigorous older man who strongly prefers the operation.

Apart from the age and health of the patient, the stage of the cancer is also a crucial factor in the choice of therapy. Surgery is most efficacious when the tumor is confined within the prostatic capsule. When it extends beyond the capsule, as in Stages C or T3, but has not yet invaded the lymph nodes, many, perhaps most, physicians believe radiation may be the better option. When metastasis has occurred, neither surgery nor radiation can effect a cure, but radiation of the pelvic area may reduce or prevent some local symptoms.[22] Irradiation by means of radioactive seed implants, often combined with external beam radiation, tends to be used on larger tumors, to make sure the radiation goes directly to the diseased area rather than to surrounding healthy tissue. It appears, however, that external beam technique has improved to the point that the use of radioactive seeds is diminishing.

Finally, of course, a given patient may simply prefer, for whatever reason, to choose irradiation over surgery. That is a legitimate option. Early on, I had wondered about whether it might be possible to undergo irradiation now and, if the cancer flared up in four or five years, to have a prostatectomy at that point. Although surgeons do occasionally perform what they call a "salvage prostatectomy," the label reflects their attitude toward it. Radiation, it seems, does such damage, particularly to blood vessels, that subsequent surgery is effectively ruled out in most cases. On the other hand, radiation can be used as a follow-up measure to surgery, as when the post-operative pathological report or a subsequent biopsy or a rising PSA level reveals that some cancerous tissue had to be left behind.

Some articles gave irradiation a more positive assessment than others, and some gave thoughtful support to watchful waiting. But even those that called it essentially a draw typically included a sentence near the end to the effect that, "Of course, for younger men in good health, surgery remains the indicated response to early stage prostatic cancer."

David Bybee had told me that Eugene Carlton liked to performed prostatectomies by the perineal approach—coming in from behind the scrotum. The fact that he said this led me to infer that there is at least one other approach, probably from the front.

I was right. I would read more in the coming days about the "nerve-sparing" version of prostatic surgery, and of Dr. Patrick Walsh's role in develop-

ing it, but I picked up some key information during my first foray. The newer operation is called a
radical retropubic prostatectomy. It is "radical"
because it involves removing the entire prostate.
"Retropubic" sounded like an approach from the
rear, but I knew that could not be correct, since
one of its advertised advantages is that, by coming in from the front through a large opening and
working behind the pubic bone—hence, retropubic—the surgeon gets a good view of the plumbing. The nerves to be spared are those that facilitate erection, and they come in two sets.
Depending on how close the tumor is to these two
"neurovascular bundles," it is often possible to let
them remain intact so that return of erections is
possible after a period of enforced leisure. The
patient's age and preoperative level of sexual
activity are important factors in predicting outcomes. Other things being equal, the younger the
man and the stronger his preoperative erections,
the better chance he has of regaining sexual function. If only one set can be spared, a man in his
forties has a decent chance of recovering erectile
capacity. A man in his mid-fifties will be much
better off if both sets can be spared. In one series
of 100 of Walsh's patients, 86 percent regained
potency within a year. In another, larger series of
600 patients operated on between 1982 and 1988,
68 percent of men who were potent before the

operation regained potency by 18 months, with the best results obtained among younger men.

A careful reader could not help noticing that, as David Bybee had indicated, the criteria for "recovery" were modest. In several studies, potency was defined as "erection sufficient for penetration and orgasm," a phrase suggestive of the tone *Consumer Reports* might take in describing the ability of a Yugo to cross the Rockies. Perhaps it could make it to the other side, but no one would confuse its performance with that of a Jaguar or Mercedes. Clearly, this smacked of Honorable Mention rather than Blue Ribbon sex. Still, there was a time in my life when "penetration and orgasm" at even the humblest level would have seemed a magnificent boon. Perhaps I could regain that adolescent sense of wonder and longing.

Dr. Walsh and a few other surgeons around the country have been performing the nerve-sparing operation for about a decade. The names that appeared most often in the materials I saw were, in addition to Walsh, William Catalona at Washington University Medical School in St. Louis, Thomas Stamey of Stanford, and Peter Scardino of Baylor. I gathered rather quickly that experience counts. As the author of one journal article put it, "There is as yet no evidence that the average urologist performs the anatomic [nerve-sparing] radical prostatectomy with outcomes comparable to those of the few centers of surgical expertise that publish results."[23]

Because of the newness and difficulty in performing the radical retropubic prostatectomy, many surgeons still use the older perineal approach in which they were trained. It is effective in treating cancer and relatively less traumatic to the patient. Because it is performed without the advantage of direct vision, however, it is also far more likely to leave a patient impotent. Based on what Dr. Bybee had told me, I assumed Dr. Carlton had, for whatever reason, not bothered to learn the new technique. I know plenty of older academics who are quite good at what they do, but have not kept up with the latest intellectual fashions. I am sometimes one of them. If that was the case with Dr. Carlton, I didn't hold it against him, but I also didn't intend to let him operate on me. As it turned out, my assumptions were entirely erroneous, but they affected my attitude and, ultimately, my actions.

I did not look forward to surgery, recognizing as I did that the quality of my life and the nature of my relationship to Patricia might well take a decided downward turn as a consequence, but those nine hours in the library had convinced me of the course I would take. With no clinical qualifications whatever, but on the basis of repeated negative DREs and ultrasound tests, I diagnosed my cancer as an A1. I decided it was about the size of a BB, a tiny BB at that, and almost certainly curable. I felt confident I was going to survive and, with a little luck, might not lose anything I would miss too much.

Late that evening, I called Patricia in Mexico City to let her know I was doing fine and to tell her that surgery definitely looked like the way to go. She observed that I sounded as if my spirits had brightened, as indeed they had. I didn't consider surgery a sure bet, but I did believe it gave me the best odds, and just getting that one settled was a relief.

CHAPTER 5

ST. PATRICK

I don't remember much about Sunday. I think I went to church, but I'm not sure. I know I spent several hours reading articles I had photocopied and I made another brief trip to the medical library to get a book I had forgotten to check out the day before. At some point, David Berg, a close friend whom we often see on weekends, called to see how we were doing. A prominent trial lawyer, David is one of the brightest and funniest people I know, with an amazing gift for lightning repartee in almost any circumstance, but he took my news quite soberly. We agreed to have dinner the next evening.

I spent Sunday evening with Rex and his wife Mary and their daughter Molly, who had just celebrated her first birthday. Like Rex, Mary is an attorney. She is also one of my heroes. Her mother died when she was quite young, her father during her first year in college. She has had some other undeserved sadnesses and some serious health problems of her own, including a probable case of cholera picked up at a restaurant. And yet, she maintains a strength and equilibrium and matter-of-fact pleasantness that sometimes defy understanding. Rex is a man of superb character and, to the best of my knowledge, has never had an enemy. Folk like that often have good babies, and as I watched Molly smear her carrots and study a plastic stack-toy and pull herself up by the rung of a chair to practice her brand-new and still imperfect talent for walking, I was aware of another powerful reason for wanting to stay alive a long time.

On Monday, I taught as best I could, but devoted most of the day to continued research. My sister had been true to her word. When I arrived at the office, the fax machine was spilling out page after page of articles she thought might prove helpful. I had already seen some of them, but some were new. Her unfailing candor and directness showed themselves in the last article to roll out: a thorough discussion, with pictures, of various forms of penile implants.

Others pitched in as well. Jim Pomerantz brought me a copy of Tom Alexander's article in *Fortune*. After making his own extensive inquiries, including interviews with a number of experienced urologists, Alexander, 62, decided to follow a course of watchful waiting but made it clear he understood it was a gamble and that not everyone would agree with his decision. About a third of the way through the article, Alexander tells of asking a urologist what he would do if he, like Alexander, had a PSA of 5.9, a suspicious ultrasound, and a positive biopsy report. Without hesitation, the urologist said he would have a radical prostatectomy. Alexander's research persuaded him that a more conservative approach was at least plausible. The article closes when Alexander's wife asks a urological surgeon who had trained under Patrick Walsh at Johns Hopkins what he would do if he were a prostate-cancer victim. His answer, which surprised Alexander, was "I honestly don't know." This article didn't change my mind, but neither did it offer great reassurance.

Fortuitously, the November issue of *The Atlantic Monthly* appeared on Monday. My own copy didn't arrive for a week, but after a couple of people mentioned that it contained a long article on prostate cancer, I went to a newsstand and picked one up. With the solidity, clarity, fairness, and moderation that consistently characterize pieces in *The Atlantic*, Charles C. Mann addressed himself primarily to the important question of whether improved and widespread screening for prostate cancer will lead millions of men to seek treatment for minor cancers that, if left alone, might cause less suffering than the treatment and at far less cost. One research team cited by Mann noted that the national medical bill for prostate cancer in

1990 was $255 million; they estimated that the cost of treatment generated by a national screening program might run as high as $28 billion—an astronomical 110-fold increase that could bankrupt Medicare or a successor national health program.

Public health implications are a critical issue, but they were not my primary concern at the moment. Three smaller segments of the story galvanized my attention more effectively. The first explained the nature of Patrick Walsh's contribution to prostatic surgery. Before Walsh, a radical prostatectomy was a particularly bloody operation, endangering the patient and preventing the surgeon from seeing what he was doing. Small wonder, then, that post-operative incontinence was common and impotence virtually certain. Incredible as it may seem to those who imagine physicians surely know where everything is and how it works, even if they can't always fix it, the orthodox view of the anatomy of the prostate was not just inadequate; it was quite mistaken.

Walsh's first breakthrough came when he located the major veins in the prostatic region and figured out how to clamp them and stop the blood flow, enabling him to see what he was cutting. That proved to be an enormous help in reducing post-operative incontinence. In men, the urinary tract has two sphincters. One of these, which women do not have, is located at the point where the bladder empties into the portion of the urethra that runs through the prostate. It operates autonomically—on its own, without conscious effort by the owner—and helps keep the semen and prostatic fluid ejaculated during orgasm from backing up into the bladder. The second sphincter, situated just millimeters from the other end of the prostate, is used to exercise conscious control over urination. When working blindly, physicians frequently destroyed both sphincters during surgery, leaving men with no effective mechanism for keeping urine from leaking out as soon as it reached the bladder. By stanching the flow of blood, Walsh was able to see well enough to leave the lower sphincter intact when he removed the prostate—unless, of course, the cancer had already spread to the sphincter. Though improvements are being made, the operation still involves loss of the upper sphincter, which is why most prostatectomy patients experience incontinence for a few weeks or months, until the external sphincter learns to take full responsibility.

Despite this advance, Walsh still assumed little could be done to spare a patient from impotence. Until 1982, urologists believed that the nerves that control erection run through the prostate. Take out the gland and the nerves go with them—wham, bam, damn. Dr. Walsh saw no reason to question that view until a patient whose prostate he had removed reported that he had regained sexual function. Since the prostate was gone but the nerves obviously were not, Walsh had to consider the possibility that the nerves did not, in fact, run through the prostate.

How could it be that such a basic anatomical arrangement was not fully understood? As Mann explained, a fully developed prostate is surrounded by fatty tissue that does not survive embalming. In the cadavers used for medical research, the gland has undergone so much deterioration that careful study is difficult. Since it was assumed that physicians already knew what they needed to know about the prostate, no one bothered to pursue the matter much further. Then, in 1981, Patrick Walsh attended a medical convention in the Netherlands. While there, he met Pieter Donker, a retired urologist who told him he had discovered that the prostates of stillborn infants, though small, are excellent subjects of study, because the fatty tissue is thin and the nerves easier to see. When Donker invited him to join him in a dissection, "Walsh observed, to his excitement, that the nerve bundles were outside the prostate capsule, held in place by a thin, almost translucent sheet called the pelvic fascia. Scalpels had been blindly cutting through them. Lifting away the fascia like a blanket from a bed would give surgeons a clear path to the prostate."[24] Using this knowledge, Walsh performed the first nerve-sparing prostatectomy in April 1982, on a fifty-two-year-old man. Within a year, the man had regained sexual function.

Over the next six years, Dr. Walsh performed more than 600 radical prostatectomies. Of these, 92 percent regained complete urinary control; 68 percent of those who were potent before the operation regained sexual function, with younger men (under sixty) doing even better. Since 1988, Walsh has performed an additional 700 radical prostatectomies. He has not as yet published data on these cases, but he has noted that his own skills have improved over time. In the meantime, William Catalona at Washington University in St. Louis, Thomas Stamey of Stanford, Peter Scardino at Baylor, and a modest number of other surgeons have achieved comparable results.

I was pleased finally to have some understanding of how the nerve-sparing technique worked. My pleasure at understanding was more than matched, however, by the terror contained in a single paragraph a few pages later. Returning to the economics of widespread screening and its inevitable aftermath of greatly increased levels of treatment, Mann observed that "although many men diagnosed as having prostate cancer will never feel any effects from the disease, failing to treat the rest would sentence thousands of people to *a death of rare awfulness.*" Mann did not use italics or boldface type. He didn't need to. I expect never to forget those last five words and the impact they made upon me. To elaborate, Mann quoted Dr. William Catalona: "Every fifteen minutes an American man dies of prostate cancer. And when that happens, he's been through hell. None of them have a pleasant death. There's a long period of pain and agony with broken bones, urinary obstruction, constipation from all the morphine—it's horrible."[25] I knew prostate cancer could kill and I assumed some pain would be involved. I had not thought in terms of "a death of rare awfulness." From that moment forward, I would.

A third memorable item in Mann's article appeared in the final paragraph. In conversation with a medical statistician whom he described as "deeply skeptical of a national screening program," Mann asked the 49-year-old researcher what he would do if he were found to have a sizable carcinoma in his prostate. To my surprise, and apparently to Mann's, the response was immediate and decisive: "Personally, I would start talking to the best surgeon I could find."[26] That seemed to me to be a good next step.

Given my assumption that Dr. Carlton did not

use the nerve-sparing technique, I expected he would refer me to someone else as soon as I told him that would be my preference. I assumed he would recommend someone at Baylor, probably Peter Scardino. My task now was to learn more about Scardino and to explore other possible options as well. I didn't know what the chances of getting access to Patrick Walsh might be, but it didn't seem out of the question. I have a good friend in the medical school at Hopkins who might be able to help, and, since my sister lives in Baltimore, it would be no problem for me to recuperate at her home for a couple of weeks. On the other hand, there was much to be said for taking care of the matter less than six blocks away.

For the next couple of days, I spent a good bit of time on the telephone, making inquiries of my own and asking others to make them for me. Since they were providing me with candid and confidential ratings of professional colleagues, I won't identify them by name, but I was profoundly aware of the value of their willingness and ability to help. A physician/administrator at a large urban hospital responded with greater than average understanding. Just a few months earlier, he had thought he was facing the same decision, until a lump in his prostate proved to be benign. Prior to getting the good news, he had decided to opt for surgery. He noted that the ideal approach

would be to practice watchful waiting for as long
as feasible, and then have the surgery.   He
acknowledged, however, that this approach could
prove fatal if one misjudged the speed of the cancer's advance. His general advice was to choose
the best doctor I could find and let him make the
decision as to the appropriate treatment. Since I
was not in a "Trust me" mood and seemed headed toward surgery, he ventured that Peter
Scardino was as good as anyone in this region, or
perhaps in the whole country. He acknowledged
that my choice was a hard one.

Another old friend, a professor in a major medical school, asked the head of urology at his institution what he would recommend. The report
was brief and clear. Radiation, he said, is less
complicated, but if he were in my place, he would
choose surgery. It isn't perfect, but the techniques
are getting better. Further, while acknowledging
that a good case can be made for watchful waiting, he favored decisive action. If he could get on
Pat Walsh's table, he said, he would be on an air-
plane in a minute. He noted, however, that Peter
Scardino is excellent, that he has "all the right
people" around him, and that members of the
Baylor staff have done the operation thousands of
times.

A Rice engineering colleague involved in biomedical research urged me not to wait too long.

"Basically," he said, "it is a race against time. These things grow slowly, but you never know when a bad cell is going to break loose, get into the blood stream, and travel to some other part of your body." He also had good things to say about Peter Scardino, who had operated successfully on a relative of his.

My friend and co-sufferer Sam, back from his conference, said that although he had decided to have his surgery done in Washington by a doctor who had trained under Walsh, he had heard so many good things about Scardino that he had seriously considered coming back to Houston just for the operation. He also told me that one of the reasons he had not already had the surgery was that he was laying in a supply of his own blood, to avoid taking a chance on contracting hepatitis or AIDS, in case he needed a transfusion. This was something I had not really considered, but it now seemed like an excellent idea.

Monday evening, David Berg and I had dinner. We joked some—when I asked if he knew Peter Scardino, he said, "He's a fine man. He's one of the mainstays of my drug and alcohol rehabilitation group"—but it was pretty serious. After listening to me talk about my fears and my quest for the perfect surgeon, he looked me dead in the eye and said, "You must promise me that you will not let money be a factor in this. You are a humble college professor. I'm not. I am offering you whatever you need to get this done right. If I were ever to find out that you had settled for something less than the very best because you didn't have the money, I would consider it a serious violation of our friendship."

I knew I would have to spend money I would prefer to keep, but I had not been too worried. My insurance would pay 80 percent and I felt fairly certain I could handle the rest without crippling strain. Still, knowing that money did not have to figure into my decision gave me an enormous feeling of freedom. I thought the chances I would ever need a penny from David were quite small. I also thought it unlikely I would ever receive many gifts I would cherish more than the one he had just given me.

Tuesday, I heard from my friend at Hopkins. He had learned that Patrick Walsh would be able to see me, but not until December, and that probably meant he could not do the surgery until January, at the earliest. He didn't think it made sense to wait. I could see one of Walsh's close colleagues the following week, but a urologist he had consulted, on learning I lived in Houston, asked why I wanted to come to Baltimore, volunteering—without my friend's mentioning the name—that "Peter Scardino at Baylor is as good as anyone at Hopkins."

Someone else told me that the former president of Turkey, the Governor of Mississippi, and Jerry Lewis had all chosen Dr. Scardino to remove their prostates. Though I don't identify closely with any of those gentlemen and might have felt more confident if Sean Connery was an alumnus of the operation, I assumed they were in a position to receive sound advice and could afford the best treatment in the world, wherever it was.

Increasingly, I began to think of Peter Scardino as a future best friend.

Patricia returned from Mexico on Tuesday evening; on Wednesday, we met with Dr. Carlton. This time, the wait was short. We sat on straight chairs about four feet from each other, against the wall. Carlton sat on a stool in the middle of the room. Once again, he was cordial, but to the point. He repeated what he had told me on the telephone: One of the biopsy samples was definitely malignant; surgery was indicated. At the time of surgery, he would remove several pelvic lymph nodes and send them to the pathology lab immediately for a quick assessment. If they were free of cancer and the gland itself showed no extension of the tumor beyond the capsule, he would proceed with the operation, giving me a 90 percent chance of cure. If examination of the capsule and the nodes indicated the tumor had

already spread, there would be no point in removing the prostate, since I could not be cured. He
would sew me back up and then I could choose
between physical or chemical castration, which
would probably keep the cancer in remission for
several years. If I chose the chemical route, he
would use a hormone called Lupron, which
would cause my libido to subside and my breasts
to swell.

I appreciate breasts as much as the next man,
but my narcissism stops short of wanting a lovely
pair of my own. "What are the chances it has
already spread?" I asked.

"18 percent," he said.

Two weeks earlier, 18 percent had sounded like
a long shot, especially for a guy with a golden
horseshoe. In the interim, I had learned that it
was quite possible for me to draw one of those 18
black beans. The despair I had temporarily managed to shelve dropped once again like a stone
through my innards. Patricia said later that my
face also fell, and that she had wanted to touch
me, but the arrangement of our chairs had made
that awkward, and she had feared that if we
looked at each other for more than a glance, both
of us would come apart.

I told Dr. Carlton I had been reading and asked
what he estimated the stage of my tumor to be,
adding hopefully, "A1?"

"A2," he said. "It's moderately differentiated."

That was one stage higher than my estimate. My BB was turning to goat cheese.

"What is my Gleason score?"

"Seven."

Remember, I had expected a three. I had also failed to note that the Gleason score is obtained by adding the grade numbers of the two most prominent patterns of cancerous tissue or, if only one pattern is present, by doubling that number. As it happens, the dominant pattern in my tumor was a three, the second most common a four. I was not far off, but in my ignorance, I thought the virulence of my tumor had just been elevated from a three to a seven. Since Dr. Carlton thought I knew what I was talking about, it didn't occur to him to straighten me out.

"Seven is the watershed score," he said. "It's moving right along, but we can usually cure it if we catch it there, before it gets to eight. That's why we need to take it out."

He went on to address the two side effects of surgery. Only three percent of his patients suffer from permanent incontinence; 70 percent regain potency within a year, if they were potent beforehand.

Recognizing that results of this magnitude were possible only with the retropubic approach, and recalling that David Bybee had told me Carlton favored the perineal approach, I asked if he used the perineal or the retropubic approach.

"I do both," he said, "but the perineal wouldn't make any sense for you." That was exactly what I thought, but it was also the reason I assumed he would not be performing my surgery. I did not want to be rude, but since this was the only prostate I would ever have, I didn't intend to let go of it carelessly.

"How many of these operations have you done?"

"Hundreds. I do four or five a week."

"How do your results compare with Dr. Scardino's?"

"The same. This is about the only operation either one of us does these days."

"I've thought about laying in a supply of blood. How many of your patients need a transfusion?"

"About one out of three."

He seemed faintly amused, but not offended, that I was questioning his credentials. I sensed he had no doubts about his competence to do as good a job as anyone else could do, but did not regard my inquiries as inappropriate. He had made my task more difficult by assuming he would be my surgeon, but he had also gone a long way toward convincing me he was up to the task. For the moment, I had no more questions.

He told me his nurse would set up an appointment for a bone scan. He assured me there was only a remote chance the cancer had already metastasized to the bones, but we might as well find out for sure. As we left the office, Janet Fuentes told me to call back the next day to find out about the bone-scan appointment. When those results came in, we could set a date for the surgery. Perhaps sensing that I had been discouraged by what the doctor had said, she gave me a brief pep talk. "It looks like there's only one really bad spot and that it's still contained in the capsule. There's a damn good chance you're going to be completely cured." I liked having Janet Fuentes on my side, but as Patricia and I walked back to our car in the parking garage, the optimism I had felt early in the week was gone. Perhaps for the first time, the possibility that this disease might actually kill me, not long after it castrated me, took a firm hold in my consciousness.

Since I was finding it difficult to concentrate on anything other than my health, I was pleased things were proceeding rapidly. I wanted to move through all the steps as quickly as possible. David Bybee had set up my second-opinion appointment for 8:30 on the following morning. The doctor I was scheduled to see was Richard Babaian, one of the two top prostate cancer specialists at the M. D. Anderson Cancer Center.

For twenty-five years, I have lived within easy walking distance of M. D. Anderson, one of the world's foremost opponents of this fearsome family of diseases. At some level, I suppose I had recognized the theoretical possibility that I might one day be a patient there, but cancer had never been one of my frontline fears. My father died of a kidney disease that probably killed his father, though diagnosis was less precise 50 years ago. My mother and four of her fourteen siblings either now have or have already died of Alzheimer's disease. I am told that gives me a 50-50 chance of the same fate. Obviously, my gene pool has some stagnant spots, but only two or three members of a quite large extended family have ever suffered from cancer not directly traceable to smoking. Since I don't smoke or work around pollutants or eat charred meat or neglect my fiber, I have long expected I would either die fairly young of kidney disease or finish out my days in a fetal position, uncomprehending of even the most basic sensations. Given the choice, I might well opt for cancer, but I had just never thought of it as part of my future. Now, I was about to be officially inducted into the Cancer Club, with all the rights and privileges pertaining thereto.

The M. D. Anderson Cancer Center is a big operation, accepting 13,500 new patients each year. Inevitably, that means a full compliment of bureaucratic procedures and their leading side effect: waiting. After signing in, I dipped into my briefcase full of prostate literature and began reading, but I couldn't help noticing my fellows-in-waiting and trying to guess at their stories. I was particularly struck by a large, ungainly woman who leaned heavily onto her equally attractive husband's shoulder. Both were dressed for weather thirty degrees colder, so I assumed they were from out of town. No native Houstonian wears heavy wool coats in October. He stared ahead stolidly. Tears streamed down her face from owlish eyes distorted further by thick glasses. I guessed she was the patient, fearing for her life, and he the awkward husband, unable to offer the succor she sought. Then I wondered if he might not be the dying one, terrified into near-stupor, while she anguished at the thought of losing the love of her life. Whichever was true, I recognized that I felt more closely akin to both of them than I would have two weeks earlier. Not everything I could learn from cancer was in my briefcase.

When my name was finally called, I went to a lab to have blood drawn and to provide a urine sample, then to a small room for a consultation with a social worker. As I got deeper into the bowels of the institution, I found the friendly, upbeat spirit my friend Frank had commended to me. A nurse talked to me about a Rice student we both knew. My "coordinator" turned out to be the wife of an Episcopal minister with whom I had recently visited. The social worker, a pleasant woman about my age, listened sympathetically and spoke realistically about the strains involved in facing the possibility of impotence and death.

I had hoped to be finished by mid-morning. At noon, my coordinator suggested I have lunch in the cafeteria and come back about two o'clock. Hundreds of people were already eating. Many were hospital personnel. Others were probably visiting relatives. Bald heads, bad wigs, and radiation templates painted on faces and necks made it obvious that some were fighting for their lives. It was almost impossible to imagine, much less acknowledge, that I belonged in this third category. Emotionally, I was mildly depressed, but physically, I felt fine. How could it be that I had a potential killer deep inside me?

Not long after I returned to the clinic area, I was ushered into a room and met by a likable young physician's assistant named Gonzalez. He ran through a long schedule of questions and, inevitably, asked me to "drop trou" and performed a DRE. He said he thought he felt something. I hoped he was wrong. He wasn't sure; the doctor could confirm or reject his finding.

Shortly after Mr. Gonzales left, I finally met

Dr. Babaian. He appeared to be a no-nonsense man, working a busy schedule, aware that this was a second-opinion visit and that we would probably never see each other again, but also committed to giving me a professional assessment of my condition. The Baylor lab had sent over my files and the slides from my biopsy. He told me the Anderson pathologists agreed with their counterparts at Baylor. Then he did a DRE. Though I now thought of myself as a veteran of DREs, he was more thorough than I had ever dreamed possible.

"I think I felt something on the right side," he said, stripping off his latex gloves. "It could be scar tissue from the biopsy, but it's probably a nodule."

"Would you think it's an A2?"

"I'd call it a B, probably a B1."

In 24 hours, my tumor had been upstaged two steps. I registered dismay.

He waved his hand dismissively. "There's not much difference between an A2 and a B when it comes to treatment." He then set out his goals and my options.

"Our three goals are survival, continence, and potency—in that order."

I respected his point of view, but my first thought was that, if I were going to be impotent, maybe I would want to piss on everybody.

KVCC KALAMAZOO VALLEY COMMUNITY COLLEGE LIBRARY

Perhaps I wasn't the first to respond in this way;
in any case, he seemed to know what I was thinking.

"Continence is an issue all the time. It's very
important."

I resisted his assertion for the moment, but
knew he was probably correct. I had read that my
kidneys manufactured at least two ounces of
urine an hour. Even when I was eighteen, my
testes couldn't match that pace.

Dr. Babaian then laid out the familiar options
for treatment. M. D. Anderson is noted for its successful use of radiation therapy, and I expected he
might make a good case for it, but he did not.
Radiation, he said, would probably offer me ten
years of survival, though I would not be disease-
free for all of that time. Over the longer term, he
estimated I would have an 85 percent chance of
living at least 15 years with surgery, compared to
a 55 percent chance with radiation. Furthermore,
he volunteered, radiation carries a greater chance
of complications, with 75 percent of patients suffering acute complications that go away fairly
quickly, but with at least 20 percent suffering serious long-term complications. These were the
worst figures on radiation I had heard. Surgery
also had its problems, he noted, but they were not
as serious. His claims for preserving potency
were comparable to those Dr. Carlton had reported,

but his figures on permanent incontinence were
less encouraging—10 percent, compared to 3 percent at Baylor. As for radiation followed by
surgery at some point down the road, he said the
complication rate is enormous, making it an
unwise course of action.

I told him that, since I had started out at Baylor,
I saw no real reason to change, which he accepted
as a matter of course. Then I asked if he would be
willing to tell me, in strict confidence, his opinion
of the relative expertise of two or three surgeons.
He smiled and said it was pointless to ask, but
that it did make sense to look for the very best.

As we prepared to end the visit, I told him I
had been feeling fairly positive until I learned that
the tumor had already spread to the lymph nodes
in 18 percent of men in my situation. He paused a
moment, then said, "That's the conventional figure, but it's too high. With the new emphasis on
screening and the PSA test, we're just not seeing
that rate. We're going to have to revise our figures. I think the chances that your lymph nodes
are involved are less than 10 percent, probably
less than 5 percent. Don't worry so much."

That helped. I felt moderately better as I left
the building and walked toward my car. I now
had no remaining doubts that I would have the
surgery, and as soon as possible. The peace I
experienced from sealing that decision did not

pass understanding, but it was tangible.   I believed I would find further peace once I settled the question of who would do the surgery. As I drove home, I decided it was time to contact Peter Scardino.

As it happens, a colleague who works with Patricia also collaborates on cancer-related research with Dr. Scardino. He had already volunteered to make inquiries on my behalf, so I asked him to find out if he could help me arrange for a consultation on short notice. Friday morning, he called to say that Pat Meyers, Dr. Scardino's nurse, would be waiting for a call from me around three o'clock that afternoon. I spent the intervening hours trying to get expert and unbiased assessments of the Drs. Carlton and Scardino. Somewhat to my surprise, I was successful. To my disappointment, it didn't help much. Every person in my sample of four, all in a position to offer trustworthy advice, gave extremely high marks to both men. "They are two of the best in the country....There are people one should not go to, but I would feel very comfortable with either one of them....I would be willing to let either one operate on me or a member of my family." Two said—quite sincerely, I believe—that they simply could not choose between them. One gave a slight edge to Gene Carlton, the other a slight edge to Peter Scardino. It seemed clear I could not make a mistake.

About four o'clock, after a round of telephone tag, I spoke to Pat Meyers. She spoke glowingly of Dr. Carlton and said he had recruited Dr. Scardino directly from his residence training at U.C.L.A. Still, if I wanted to talk with Dr. Scardino, she could work me in at 10:00 A.M. on the following Wednesday. She could see Patricia and me the afternoon before, to address some common questions ahead of time. I asked her about my chances of getting on Dr. Scardino's schedule if I decided I wanted him to do the surgery. His schedule was crowded, she said, but it could be arranged. Her voice was soothing and kind, but her ear was even better. She said, "Mr. Martin, you sound so worried."

I told her I was indeed frightened, particularly at hearing there was an 18-percent chance the cancer had already spread to the lymph nodes. (I hadn't forgotten Dr. Babaian's skepticism regarding that figure, but I had reverted to believing the worst.) "You're being too pessimistic," she said. "You need to come talk to me." Scientific medicine is a marvelous achievement, but the healing touch—physical, verbal, or simply present in one's expression and manner—is a balm suffused with restorative power. By the time we finished talking, a peaceful confidence began to well up within me and warm my heart, because I knew that, somehow, Pat Meyers was going to see to it that I got well.

Without knowing precisely why or being able to provide a clear rationale, I decided I would ask Peter Scardino to perform my surgery. Reaching that decision and recognizing I had reached it seemed to lift a burden. I called David Bybee to tell him I was thinking seriously of switching to Peter Scardino, for reasons hard to explain. He reasserted his strong confidence in Gene Carlton, but acknowledged that Scardino was excellent. "A doctor is concerned that you be happy and comfortable and that you get good care. It's no problem. I'll arrange it." I'm not convinced every doctor subscribes to this idealistic view, but I believe David Bybee does, and that is a major reason he holds an executive position on my health-management team.

That evening, Patricia and I went to Carabbas, a popular Italian restaurant, and I ordered a marvelous bowl of fettucine Alfredo topped with goat cheese, red peppers, and grilled chicken. As I recall, we had some wine. We ate and drank and laughed and talked as we had not for ten days. I had bad moments and anxious spells after that evening, but never again any to match those that had gone before. That devilish little tumor gnawing away inside me didn't know it yet, but the healing had already begun.

Early Saturday, we made the three-hour drive to Wimberley, where we were wrapping up construction of our new home. An implausible series of maddening delays, most of which were attributable to a contractor whose personal and organizational imperfections forced him into bankruptcy and us into substantial unexpected debt, had turned the dream of a decade into a protracted nightmare. Still, the workmanship on the house was excellent, the design exceeded our high expectations, and we loved sitting on the porch and looking west out to the point where the earth curved out of sight. Best of all, it was finally finished. All that remained was wrapping up the paperwork and writing checks to anyone who happened to be standing around the office at the title company.

October is probably Texas's most agreeable month, and a clear sky and full moon brought a cool, crisp day to perfection. At dusk, we drove the pickup out to Fischer for the annual Harvest Moon Ball, sponsored by the Wimberley Institute of Cultures—both appellations quite consciously overblown. On the way, a country-music station from Austin played a song whose message was, "If you love her, don't forget to hold her sometime other than at night." This was not the first time I had heard that sentiment expressed. I smiled and looked at Patricia, who seemed to be growing more beautiful every day. "That's probably good advice." I allowed. She returned my smile with warm recognition. "Could be," she said.

Fischer Hall and a long, narrow building that houses a four-lane members-only bowling alley on the same plot of ground are all that remain of what was never more than a tiny settlement of German farmers and ranchers. The hall, a picturesque barnlike structure with wooden flaps that can be propped open to catch the breeze, has been well-preserved and must look much like it did a century ago, when the folk attending a harvest dance had actually been harvesting. The dance was preceded by a fajita dinner served on long wooden tables outside the hall underneath a brilliant, full harvest moon whose light was supplemented by kerosene lanterns. The folk at our table were, like us, refugees from the city in search of clean air, quiet, low humidity, and minimum hassle. Most of them had retired to Wimberley several years earlier and spoke glowingly of watching sunsets, fishing, playing golf, painting, or just piddling around. I wasn't ready to retire and I didn't want to trade pastimes with them, but they seemed genuinely happy with their lives and each other. Later, as Patricia and I waltzed and two-stepped and danced the polka and the Schottisch and the Cotton-Eyed Joe to the oompah strains of Roy Haag and his Bohemian Dutchmen, I could not suppress an aching desire to live a long, long time, and to hold my lover lots of times other than at night.

CHAPTER 6

St. Peter

On Tuesday morning at eight, I pedaled over to
Methodist Hospital for the first part of the bone-
scan procedure. On seeing my helmet, the technician chuckled and said he could not remember
ever having had a patient ride a bike to his bone-
scan appointment. He injected a radioactive substance into a vein in my arm and told me to come
back in three hours. I went on to Rice and attended a long committee meeting, then returned at
eleven for the scan itself. During those three
hours, the substance had moved through my
bloodstream looking for a home. When a bone
suffers damage, whether from arthritis, a fracture,
or cancer, the body tries to repair itself by producing new bone. The new bone, still not fully hardened, will absorb the isotope. As I stood or lay
down upon a table, a large machine that operates
something like a Geiger counter was passed in
turn over all parts of my body, in search of sites
where concentrations of radioactive isotope
would indicate the presence of bones under
repair. In the absence of any known arthritis or
fractures, and in the presence of a positive biopsy,

any hot spots it found would be a strong sign my cancer had already spread.

The room was cool and the machine brought to mind stories of people dragooned into UFOs by aliens and subjected to involuntary exploration of their bodies, but the procedure itself was so simple and peaceful that I went to sleep on the table, causing the technician some momentary concern. As is usual in medical labs, he gave no indication as to what he was seeing, but I knew that the chances I already had bone cancer were exceedingly remote, and that the main purpose of the test was to establish a benchmark, so that any scans I had in future years could be compared to this one to see if unexplained changes had taken place. I was truly not worried, and awareness of that gave me comfort.

I was scheduled to see Pat Meyers on Tuesday afternoon. I didn't think it was necessary for Patricia to go with me, but she insisted. "I want them to understand how important this is to me," she said. It's hard to counter an argument like that.

Pat Meyers proved to be as reassuring in person as she had been over the telephone. First, she showed us a medical illustration of the prostate and explained how the disease spreads and what the surgery would do. She noted that the gland has three layers of "rind." Obviously, it is best if the tumor is confined within the first layer, but as long as it does not escape the third, the chances are good that a complete cure can be effected by surgery.

Continuing, she pointed out the two sphincters at the top and bottom of the prostate and confirmed that the top one had to go. She assured me, however, that there was little reason for me to worry about incontinence. The small percentage of men who are permanently incontinent after a properly performed prostatectomy comprises, with few exceptions, those who are quite old or obese or who suffer from Parkinson's Disease or other maladies that diminish their ability to exercise control over their urinary sphincters, as well as those whose late-stage tumor has spread so far that both sphincters have to be removed. Surgical incompetence, of course, could account for another category, but that was not an issue in this office. I was almost certain to regain complete continence after a period of recovery that might last between a few days and a year. During that period, I would have to wear some kind of absorbent padding, moving in stages from adult diapers to less intrusive products, one of which resembles a sock made from a feminine hygiene napkin.

Life does have its circular ironies. As a prepubescent youth, enveloped by the darkness of the tiny Majestic Theater in Devine, Texas, I thrilled quietly at June Allyson's terminally wholesome smile and the hoarse sweetness of her voice. And now, I fantasized, she and I could run slow-motion through the meadow, gaily colored diaper bags slung over our shoulders in devil-may-care fashion. This new bond between us, however, would be but temporary. Pat explained that even if, for some reason, I did not regain virtually complete continence within a year or two, I need not be confined to adult diapers for the rest of my life. Biomedical technicians at Baylor and Methodist have developed an artificial sphincter implant, a little contraption with a manually operated spigot that works about the way it sounds like it would work.

Since I would soon be entirely dependent upon my urethral sphincter, I would need to get it into shape by doing regular sets of what are called Kegel exercises. These consist of contracting the sphincter. If you don't know where it is, you can locate it by cutting off the flow while urinating. Those are the muscles that need to be strengthened and toned up. The exercises, which should be performed several times a day, include a set of quick contractions, a second set of identical contractions lasting five seconds followed by five seconds of relaxation, and a third, slightly different, type in which the muscles are tensed as if trying to draw the entire sphincter region up into the body. One starts by doing a few repetitions in each set, then increasing the number to as many as 200 of each type. If I had difficulty with these exercises, Pat volunteered, biofeedback therapists would be available to assist me. (In fact, I have found them to be quite easy, and a time-management program on my computer still reminds me to perform them every four hours. Driving also offers good opportunities to practice; since I listen to talk shows, sphincter contraction often seems appropriate.)

While I was learning the new system, and even afterward, I would need to be careful about mounting too great a challenge for my Lone Ranger sphincter. Caffeine and carbonated beverages could stimulate it beyond its capacity to respond, and alcohol could lull it into careless relaxation. Tiredness or stress could reduce its tensile strength. The feeling of an urgent need to urinate would probably be less intense than I had been experiencing for several years, but when the need arose, my control over it would also be lessened. Therefore, I should develop the habit of relieving myself before the urge grew strong. Pat recommended that I follow a course of "timed voidings," beginning at 90-minute intervals and working up to two-and-a-half-hour intervals. Since 90 minutes was quite a stretch for me now, I didn't think I would have any trouble remembering to keep such a schedule.

Next, we talked about sex. This had loomed as a major issue from the beginning. I assume that no one reading this book has a strong interest in our sex life, and I feel no strong compulsion to provide many details. Still, when asked occasionally about what have been the key factors that have held us together for 36 years, we have always acknowledged to ourselves, and sometimes to others, that the importance of extraordinarily satisfying sexual communication would be hard to discount. We read the complaints in Ann Landers about husbands who have lost interest in sex, or wives who have never found any pleasure in it, or couples who profess to be perfectly happy although they have not made love in twenty years, and we tell each other how pleased we are that these are not our stories. When we scan the Sunday-supplement statistics on lovemaking frequency, sorted into percentiles by age groups, we smile and note that, according to the charts, we shall probably be smiling for some time to come. And, in more reflective moments, we acknowledge that we might not have made it through some rough periods in our marriage had it not been for the fact that, even when we were angry at or extremely disappointed in the other, we regularly managed to call an enthusiastic truce at bedtime. A marriage counselor once told us this pattern was rather unusual. He also told us it didn't sound like the behavior of people who were tired of each other. We concluded he was right.

In short, if it's not too late for that, the loss of the capacity for sexual intercourse was a disheartening prospect. We did not doubt that "love will find a way." Patricia repeatedly told me that the most important thing was for me to get well, but neither of us pretended our lives would be quite the same without the acts of congress that had brought us so much pleasure.

We told Pat of our keen interest in a positive outcome. "We don't want you to give up anything," she said. "We want you to have it all." To begin, she answered two crucial questions. The nerves that control erection are a completely different set from those affecting sensation, and the operation would have no physiological effect on my libido or sensation of orgasm. I had already decided I would rather feel horny and frustrated than simply lie placidly on the couch like a neutered cat. Patricia had concurred, noting that I had been horny and frustrated when we began dating in 1957, and that she had found it appealing; perhaps she could again. Fortunately, the frustration would not be terminal. Even though I would no longer produce any ejaculate, I would still be able to achieve orgasm, and it would feel much the same as before. I had assumed as much, but it was a relief to get confirmation.

From that hopeful beginning, Pat ran through the statistics for recovery of potency, and then addressed the question of what could be done if all did not go as hoped. One possibility is a vacuum device that looks something like a cross between a ray gun and a salad-shooter. The penis is inserted into a tube—an unnecessarily large tube, I thought—and a suction is produced by squeezing the trigger of a pistol-grip device. This stimulates blood flow and produces an erection, which is then maintained by a rubber pressure ring clamped around the base of the penis. I didn't want to make any sweeping statements about what I would or would not be willing to use to facilitate satisfactory sex, but this gave me another reason to be grateful for a marriage of long standing. If a woman was going to laugh at me in bed, it might help if I knew her really well.

Another possibility Pat described was injection of papavarin, a dilating chemical that causes the corpora cavernosa, two tubes of spongy tissue that run the length of the penis on each side of the urethra, to fill with blood and produce an erection. The chemical, mixed with saline and other substances, is injected right into the side of the penis near the base. Frequent use over an extended period of time can cause some problems, mainly the development of scar tissue from the needle and a build-up of plaque that can produce a curvature in the erect penis. Moderate use, however, is safe and effective. Some men balk at the idea of sticking a needle into their penis, but there are few nerves in the recommended injection site, and it is not a painful procedure. Wives, Pat said, tend to think it is great, since it produces a firm erection that typically lasts for an hour or more. I made an indelible mental note of this. Even if it turned out that my biopsy report had been a mistake, this was something to put in the file marked, "Enjoying the Golden Years." Now that I would no longer produce any ejaculate, I might even be able to fake an orgasm.

Ms. Meyers then told me what to expect with regard to the actual surgical procedure. The surgery itself would take about two-and-a-half hours, but I would be in the operating room for three-and-a-half hours, part of which would be spent waiting for the pathology report on the tissue taken from my lymph nodes. Once again, I asked about the chances the cancer would have spread to the nodes. Her answer resolved the contradictions I had heard. As Dr. Babaian had said, the 18-percent figure commonly cited is based on studies that include all patients judged to have an A or T1 tumor. Among Dr. Scardino's patients, that figure would apply only to those with PSA scores considerably higher than mine. It was quite rare, she said, to find lymph-node involvement in anyone with a PSA of less than 20. In fact, of the last 50 of Dr. Scardino's patients with numbers like mine, the lymph nodes had been clear in every single one. With a score of only 8, I could relax.

But what about my Gleason score of 7? That, too, she assured me, was not as serious as it might sound. Most of the cancerous cells were grade 3; a few were grade 4. "We consider finding a tumor while it is in the 4-7 range to be early detection."

After the operation, Pat explained, I would remain in the hospital for about a week, and then be limited in what I could do for at least two more weeks. During that time, I should sit with my legs elevated, to avoid getting a blood clot. It would be fine to walk, but I shouldn't stand still for any significant length of time—again, to avoid a blood clot. My bottom would be sore and my scrotum would swell, but the main irritant was likely to be the catheter that I would wear for three weeks. It would not be painful, but almost everyone finds it annoying. Because pulling it loose would cause serious problems, I should not drive until it was removed. Once the catheter was out, I could resume a normal schedule as soon as I felt like it, which she estimated would take about six weeks. The only restrictions would be that I should not lift anything that weighed more than ten pounds for at least 6-8 weeks, and I should refrain from any serious sexual activity, even if I were capable of it.

By now, I was ready to get on with it. How long would I have to wait? Officially, she said, Dr. Scardino's schedule was full, but he could work me in on one of three days in November: the 4th, the 15th, or the 29th. All were possible; none was ideal. Since my spirits were good, I liked the idea of moving as rapidly as possible, but I was scheduled to host a visitor from Cambridge University for ten days beginning October 30, four days away. I could get out of it, but it would be awkward. The early date also meant I would have to arrange to have my classes covered for an entire month. The 15th was fine with me, but Dr. Scardino would be leaving for Sicily the next day. If any complications arose, someone else would have to take care of them. The 29th would fall at the beginning of the last week of classes, making substitute arrangements easy, and, because it was more than a month away, I would have time to lay in a supply of blood, something the two earlier dates would not allow. On the negative side, I would still be weak at Christmas and, perhaps more pertinent, waiting too long might cause me to lapse back into depression.

Considering all the options, I was leaning toward November 4th, mainly because I did not want to take a chance, however remote, that some killer cell would break loose and set up shop in a vulnerable part of my body. Pat thought I didn't need to worry about the difference two or three weeks would make and recommended I select one of the last two dates. She seemed to favor the 29th over the 15th, primarily because Dr. Scardino would be leaving the country, but suggested I ask him if he had a preference.

On Wednesday, we met with Peter Scardino. In his late forties, but looking younger, he was tall, handsome, and smooth. He was also impressively pleasant and gracious. Pat Meyers had told us he was rushed, but he conveyed the impression that he was willing to spend whatever time was needed to answer any questions I might have. He checked to see if we had any questions about what Pat had told us.

We told him of our concern about sexual function. He was not surprised, and like his nurse, he offered a hopeful message: "Our goal is for sex to be as rich as ever for you. It may not be quite the same, but it's not the same now as it was when you were 18. That doesn't mean it can't be just as rich and satisfying." He told me I would have to lie low for at least six weeks after the operation, to avoid possible damage to my reconstructed urethra, and I shouldn't expect too much for some

time after that, "but we think it's important to stay
with it." At about three months, unless my recovery was unexpectedly remarkable, he would want
me to begin using the papavarin injections. Most
of the problems with the solution had been
worked out, so that scarring is no longer much of
a threat. He offered one caution: because the
drug typically produces an erection defiant of
time and contemptuous of gravity, some elated
men become excessively enthusiastic and use it
more than once a day. Such imprudence, he
warned, compounds the dilating effect of the drug
and can result in "priapism"—a condition named
for the Greek god of procreation and character-
ized by an erection that will not go down for
hours and hours and hours. It also hurts.
Fortunately, it can be cured by having a physician
administer an antidote. It this should happen to
me, I could call the clinic's 24-hour number and
arrange to meet a doctor. If it happened while I
was out of town, any emergency room would
have what I needed. I like to think of myself as
only moderately concerned with appearances, but
the mental image of showing up at a hospital in
the middle of the night, hat hanging on my lap,
was enough to convince me that one shot a day
would be sufficient. If we have to cut back, we'll
cut back.

Next, we talked about blood. My friend at

Johns Hopkins had ventured that "the blood supply is pretty clean; I wouldn't worry about it." In
my first conversation with Pat Meyers, she had
also defended the purity of the current supply,
volunteering that she would not bank blood if she
were having surgery, nor would she recommend
that a member of her family do so. "Fifteen years
ago, definitely. Today, with all the screens in
place, it's a wholly different situation. But if it
would give you peace of mind, it's no problem to
arrange it." Dr. Bybee had confirmed that the
chances of getting AIDS from a transfusion were
now no greater than one in a million, and those
for hepatitis about one in 500,000. He conceded,
however, that he would probably feel safer with
some of his own blood in reserve.

Dr. Scardino gave me a pamphlet containing
precise instructions for arranging an "autologous"
blood donation. Making it clear that the choice
was up to me, he also made it clear that he
thought it was an unnecessary procedure. An
otherwise healthy patient can handle the loss of
1500 ccs (three units) of blood, the standard
amount collected in autologous donations for
prostatectomies. The average loss in his surgeries
is less than 750 ccs. He noted that only one in ten
of his patients ever require a transfusion—a figure
I knew to be excellent—and most of those are men
who have rendered themselves anemic by donat-

ing their blood. This figure was based on data at least a year old at the time. A more recent assessment has revealed that the transfusion rate for Scardino's prostatectomy patients has dropped to approximately one in twenty-five operations. Of the few men who have not given blood ahead of time and still need a transfusion, most have such severe blood loss that they need more than three units and thus have to draw on the general blood supply anyway. In short, though laying in a supply of my own blood might make me feel safer, it was not likely to serve any other worthy purpose.

We had covered most of the ground and I was about to raise the issue of switching doctors when he brought it up himself. He explained that Gene Carlton had been his mentor, that they still worked as close partners, and that he had complete confidence in Dr. Carlton's ability as a surgeon. It was not uncommon for either of them to pass patients to the other, because of scheduling or simply because some patients might feel more comfortable with one than with the other. He would accept me as a patient, but he felt I would need to communicate my decision to Dr. Carlton myself. Even though Dr. Bybee had told me he would handle the transfer, I had already resolved to do this, so this was no added burden.

Now that he was officially my urologist and not just a consulting physician, Dr. Scardino felt he had earned the right to stick his finger in my rectum. Pat and Patricia stepped out the room, I removed my trousers and shorts, and the good doctor digitized me. He was not as thorough as Dr. Babaian had been, for which I was grateful. With a satisfied smile, he said he didn't think he had felt anything. If there was a bump, as Dr. Babaian had reported, it could easily have been caused by the biopsy. In any case, he was prepared to call this one a T1c tumor—undetectable except by needle biopsy. "We're seeing this more often, mainly because of the PSA test. Before [the widespread use of the test], it would have grown and we would have found it when there was a 50-50 chance of curing it. Now, we've got a 95 percent chance."[27]

Just as I was about to ask if he saw any reason for me to favor one of the three possible surgery dates over the others, Pat Meyers came in to tell him he had a telephone call. While we waited for him to return, she gave me two short videos about prostate cancer. After a few minutes, she checked to make sure he was coming back, only to discover that he, apparently unaware I had another question, had left. I was disappointed, but ready to make a decision. As I rehearsed the pros and cons of each day, she said, "We still have some more tests to do. Come back on the 4th for those and we can talk about it then."

"But the 4th is one of my choices," I protested.

"Yes," she said, with a slight smile. "That's too soon. You won't have time to get ready."

"I'd hate to wait too long."

She shook her head gently. "You're not going to wait too long."

"You're sure?"

"I'm sure."

Then what about the 15th? How important was it for the doctor to be on hand in the days following the surgery? If something had to be redone, who would do it?

Pat admitted she would probably feel uneasy about having her surgeon leave town the day after operating on her. Still, she said with a wry smile, none of the standard complications—infection, bleeding, a blood clot, or trouble with the catheter—would call for a new chapter in a medical textbook. Scardino's colleagues and a team of skilled residents would almost certainly be able to handle any trouble that might arise.

She mentioned one other possibility: Someone might cancel, opening up a more favorable date.

"How likely is that?"

"Not very. By the time people decide to have the surgery and then get on his schedule, not many of them cancel." I don't think she told me this to make a point, but it reminded me that I had broken in line and should be grateful for the choices I had. After extracting an assurance that the stated options would still be available on the 4th, we left. On the way out, I checked Dr. Carlton's office, but he was gone. When I missed him again on the 4th, I wrote him a letter, thanking him for his concern and advice, and explaining that I had no good explanation for my decision. I should have tracked him down and told him in person. We don't always do what we should.

Patricia was taken with both Pat Meyers and Peter Scardino. She appreciated the time and attention they had given and felt reassured by what she had heard. That's why it surprised me late that evening when, for the first time, she broke into sobs shortly after we lay down together in bed. "I'll be OK," she said. "I just keep thinking about when our bodies were so young and fine. When we make love, I imagine they still are. It's hard to think about losing that. But even if it all comes back this time, I know that some day one of us is going to have to face the other's infirmity. Maybe both at the same time. Of course, I've known that would happen eventually, but it's starting earlier than I had expected."

Patricia has always been sensitive to the passage of eras. As a child, she cried on her birthdays, not because she was tired or filled with sweets or disappointed about her gifts, but because she recognized she would never again be the age from which she had just graduated. In the years since childhood, other transitions—marriage, moving, a tubal ligation, sending the last child off to college, and sundry lesser moments—have generated similar reactions. I held her for a while and tried to comfort her, but I was bone-tired and finally told her I just had to go to sleep. She said it was okay and sounded as if she meant it. She stopped crying and lay there for awhile, then kissed me and went to another room, probably to watch the weather channel. She felt better the next morning. That's one of the best things about mornings.

CHAPTER 7

COMMUNITY

With my plans now firm except for the actual date of the surgery, I saw no reason not to tell a wider range of people about my condition. I wanted particularly to say something to my students. I had been teaching on automatic pilot since returning from California, and I felt bad about that. I won't pretend that I never recycle a lecture, but I do constantly add and delete and revise, so that probably a third of every course I teach is new material. For the previous two weeks, I had simply reached in the file, glanced over last year's notes, and waded through the hour as best I could. I didn't feel terribly guilty, under the circumstances, but I knew I was giving less than they deserved and, just in case they had noticed, I wanted them to know why.

I also wanted to tell them because they are my friends. Perhaps because I taught at a New England boarding school for girls when I was in my mid-twenties, I became comfortable quite early with the line that separates teachers and students. I have never tried to be a "buddy" to my students or subscribed to the notion, so popular in the Sixties and early Seventies, that I had more to learn from them than they from me. Still, I do genuinely like them, most of them anyway, and I think they know that. I make a point of learning their names, which makes the experience better for all of us. I don't want to spend four months talking to a roomful of strangers, and I suspect it induces them to perform better.

Due to administrative responsibilities, I was teaching only one large class, Introduction to Sociology, and it had already suffered a trauma. On the preceding weekend, a shy student who had the highest grade in this class, and A's in all his others, had jumped from a tower after a campus party, ending his promising young life. I nearly always begin the introductory course by talking about suicide, a much-studied phenomenon that offers excellent opportunity to compare various sociological approaches. At the end of that discussion, I tell students what to look for in themselves and others and what kind of help is available for those who may find life so oppressive as to seem unbearable. I stress particularly that they should take all talk of suicide seriously and that, if they ever feel themselves being drawn into such a vortex of misery, they should not only seek professional help, but should also remember a crucial truth about even the most serious depression: *"You will feel better.* Perhaps not soon, and perhaps not without subsequent relapse, but that, too, will pass. As unbelievable as it may seem, as miserable as you may feel, the time will come when *you will feel better!*"

I had no reason to suspect this student was contemplating suicide. On the day before his death, he asked me to look over a test on which he thought a grader had been too harsh. Surely that would indicate he intended to finish the semester. And then he was gone. I felt no real personal responsibility for his death, but I was saddened that my exhortation had not persuaded him to endure until his season of pain passed. I talked for a few minutes at the beginning of class about the loss, reminded them again of available sources of help, and stressed as strongly as I could that even the most debilitating bouts of depression can be overcome. And then I talked to them about social stratification. For the first time since my diagnosis, teaching felt good again.

With about ten minutes remaining in the period, I found a convenient stopping place and told them I had another serious something to talk about. I told them much the same things I had told my sons and daughter. I had cancer, it was operable, there was strong reason for optimism, I would not finish the semester but they would be left in good hands, and I expected to be back in harness in January. I apologized for any noticeable letdown in my teaching and told them I thought I would do better the rest of the way. I also told them that, although I knew little about many of them other than their names and their test scores, they were important to me, standing as they did for all the young people I had been privileged to teach in my 25 years at this wonderful university. The room was quite still. I saw a few tears, and so did they. When I finished, several came to the front to give me some encouragement. One of them, J.P., asked if he might come by my office some time. He said he would like to tell me something that might help. I told him I was in most afternoons, including that one.

About half an hour later, J.P. showed up. We had never talked and my main impression of him was that he bore the marks of membership in what my son Rex calls the Lucky Sperm Club—a handsome face, a brilliant smile, a winsome manner, and good taste in clothes. It was hard not to assume that almost everything had gone well in his life. And then he told me his story. While on vacation between his junior and senior years in high school, he had been stricken with terrible headaches and vision problems that would not abate. After seeing a series of doctors, he learned that he had a golf ball–sized tumor on his brain. Specialists judged the tumor could not be removed surgically and recommended irradiation as the only feasible treatment option. The prognosis was grim, but the malignant mass began to shrink and the symptoms subsided. Now, three years later, the tumor has virtually disappeared and the chances are excellent that J.P. has won. Clearly, his problem had been worse than mine, but that was not his point. Before this happened to him, he said, he had sailed through life without adequately appreciating what he had or what was going on around him. Staring death in the teeth at age eighteen had changed that. "If something like this had to happen," he said, "I'm glad it happened when I was young. I know my life will always be richer for it. You will find the same thing. This can be really important for you, in a good way."

On some days, I do learn more from my students than they learn from me.

In the afternoons that followed, other students dropped in to offer comfort and hope. Eighteen months earlier, Jennifer's father had been found to have extensive liver cancer and told he had four months to live. He is still alive. Stella's mother had lymphoma and Tandy's had breast cancer. Both had survived. Gali brought me two candles she had made and insisted, "You are going to get well!" David came by to say he was pulling for me. Emily, to whom I had never spoken directly, was standing in the outer office looking in another direction when I walked in after a meeting. When I greeted her, she looked at me and, perhaps not knowing just what to say, simply threw her arms around me and hugged me. Catherine walked by while I was standing at the elevator. Her eyes brimming with tears, she mouthed, "I'm so sorry," and rushed out of the building. Lee and Larycia and Charles all told me they would be praying for me, as did the members of the Baptist Student Union.

Many people promised to remember me in their prayers. I regard myself as a Christian, though my faith is a cyclical performer and seldom ventures far into orthodox territory these days. But even as a youth, the strictly rationalistic Fundamentalist church in which I was reared had little room for miracles. Such signs and wonders, we were told, had passed away with the death of the apostles and the closing of the Biblical canon. We prayed that God would guide the heads and hands of attending physicians and that the sick would be "restored to their normal or much-wanted health," but we expected nothing more than a modest boost to standard medical procedures and natural healing processes, and we hooted at the ranting, sweaty revivalists who claimed a gift from God that could cause the lame to walk and the blind to see. An adult lifetime spent toiling in the vineyards of sociology had not further enhanced my openness to the notion that God was likely to interrupt the web of nature to do something special for me, any more than I regarded my affliction as divine retribution for some unforgiven sin. Still, I gratefully accepted all prayers anyone wanted to offer on my behalf. I had read of a study indicating that intercessory prayer helps people get well, even when they do not know someone else is praying for them. The evidence is even stronger that individuals who feel they are part of a supportive community have a better chance of surviving cancer than those who face it alone. I had no desire to disprove either of these contentions.

Not everyone who wished me well promised to pray for me. Some said, "I'll be thinking about you" or "I'll be sending warm thoughts your way." One or two even mentioned positive vibrations. Another gave me the name of a therapist who has helped cancer and AIDS patients by teaching them to meditate. Several recommended that I read books by Bernie Siegel, an M.D. whose uplifting bestsellers are said to have helped multitudes of desperately ill people get well. I bought *Peace, Love, and Healing—Bodymind Communication & the Path to Self-Healing: An Exploration*, which I had been told was his best book, and I fully intended to read it. I still might.

I do not doubt that state of mind can cause people to get sick or help them recover, and if I were to learn that my cancer had metastasized, I would explore the "bodymind" connection more fully. For the present, however, I regarded my problem as more technical than spiritual. That outlook notwithstanding, I deeply appreciated every offer of goodwill and support, however it was framed.

Perhaps the most memorable expression of well-wishing came from the plumber/electrician who had done the work on our house in Wimberley. Britt has a problem with promptness that frustrated us mightily at times. Still, he's a talented tradesman, he's good-hearted, and when he finally shows up, it's hard to stay mad at him. He had heard about my cancer from Curlo and Margie, our neighbors up on the ridge, and he felt he ought to say something. I was sitting on the stairs that lead up to my writing room, watching him install a washing machine. As an authentic good old boy, he's not usually timid about saying whatever is on his mind, but this was a challenge for him. "I'm not no religious freak," he began. "Not by no means. But I want you to know that if I...." He looked out the window. "I mean, I'm going to...." He looked up and then down. He looked everywhere but right at me and kept on hemming and hawing. "Well, we both know that the Guy Up There who decides these things...." It was clear that Britt thought he ought to pray for me, but that his prayer life was in hiatus just now, and he didn't want to make any pledges he might not keep.

"Britt," I interrupted, "if you don't pray much these days, it's okay. I've looked into this carefully and I'm counting more heavily on my surgeon than I am on miracles."

"That's exactly the way I feel," he said, his voice regaining its heartiness.

"But," I assured him, "I appreciate your good wishes."

He stepped toward me, shook my hand warmly, looked me in the eye, and said, "You got those, Buddy. You can count on it."

As Don McNeill used to say at prayer time on the "Breakfast Club" radio program, "Each in his own words, each in his own way."

I also found unspoken strength from the example of others. I was serving on an ad hoc committee in charge of arrangements for the inauguration of Rice's new president, Malcolm Gillis. One of the members of the committee has struggled with a truly life-threatening cancer for years. It had taken a turn for the worse and her chemotherapy treatments forced her to miss several meetings. But when she was present, she talked at length about invitations and programs and luncheons, in obvious command of a myriad of details and treating them as important. Perhaps she had learned to cope by acting as if her life were not in serious peril. Perhaps I could develop the same ability. Or perhaps she was just stronger than I was. In any case, my own inability to concentrate on much of anything other than setting a date for surgery reaffirmed my conviction that I was not a suitable candidate for watchful waiting.

Another colleague, the dean of our school of music, was found to have extensive carcinoma of the pancreas about five years ago. The survival rate for that brand of cancer is approximately two percent. And yet, after exploratory surgery, a regimen of chemotherapy to shrink the tumor, a twelve-hour operation that included intra-operative radiation, subsequent surgery to install a shunt, and still more radiation, he returned to work, oversaw construction of a mammoth building to house his school, and continued to strengthen an already first-rate collection of faculty and students. The cancer has not recurred. An unusually reflective and eloquent man, he has thought of writing about his own ordeal, but is waiting until he feels more sure he is out of danger. That means all his notable accomplishments of the last several years have been forged in the constant shadow of death. I hoped that, if my cancer had already spread, I could face a clouded future with comparable grace.

I also received invaluable support from Sam,

who provided me with regular reports on his own situation. I knew when his surgery was scheduled and rejoiced to come in one afternoon and hear his wife Priscilla's voice on the answering machine, telling us his lymph nodes had been clear and the operation an apparent success. The next morning I talked to both of them on the telephone, and within a few days Sam was sending me daily e-mail reports of his progress, giving me a valuable preview of what I could expect. The pain was not bad, the catheter required conscious attention before moving, and he was eager to leave the hospital, but, overall, he was in good spirits and said nothing that made me doubt my own ability to cope with the surgery and recovery period. I had seldom been more grateful for the Internet.

One form of unexpected spirit-lifting came from women. I have never made a list of my inner circle of friends, but if I were to, I am confident that women would be at least as well represented as men. It did not surprise me that my women friends were distressed to learn I had cancer, but I was, shall we say, positively affected by the response of several. They are all middle-aged and intelligent and informed enough to understand the possible effects of prostate cancer and its treatment. Thus, when they offered observations and reported ruminations they had never before shared with me, I felt renewed appreciation for their friendship. I also felt confident they fully expected me to understand that they were ministering to the sick and afflicted, not saying anything I should take too seriously. There is safety in numbness.

Some friends, perhaps not entirely of their own choosing, helped simply by listening. A sister-in-law, Mary Ellen, called one morning to say that one of the best things a person who has received bad news can do is to tell the whole story to at least six people a week. She was offering to fill one of those spots during any week I chose. My literary agent and friend, Gerry McCauley, whose twin brother had died of cancer two years earlier and who stays in almost daily contact with the poet Donald Hall, another cancer-stricken client, checked frequently to see how I was holding up.

Others gave similar gifts. George Rupp, former president of Rice and now president of Columbia, returned with his wife Nancy to receive an award at Rice's Homecoming. While Nancy visited with Patricia and members of a reading group, George and I went to dinner. I gave him a none-too-brief summary and then tried to turn the conversation to his new post at Columbia. He brushed this aside with a slight gesture and a dismissive remark to the effect that, "It's a university. We can talk about that some other time. I want to hear about you."

I soon recognized that, perverse as it might seem, I rather enjoyed having people feel sorry for me. When, as happened on several occasions, I managed to work into conversation the fact that I had prostate cancer and the person so informed noted that his father or uncle or half a dozen of his friends had had it for years and were doing just fine, I felt cheated. I considered cultivating a sad, faraway look and telling people only that I had cancer, without specifying what kind or how advanced it was, giving them opportunity to think the worst and react appropriately.

My various conversations—many of which were initiated by friends who had gotten the news from others and did not involve strangers button-holed in hallways, gave me some interesting insights into male sexuality. Several men in my general age group seemed surprised I was wor-ried about sexual function, offering the consola-tion that, "Well, at our age, that's not much of a concern." Others seemed amazed that I would even mention the infirmity that dares not speak its name. A woman friend told of discussing my sit-uation with a mutual male friend, one of whose closest friends had undergone a prostatectomy. During several pre-operational conversations and hospital visits, neither of them had ever whis-pered the word "impotence," and, our friend admitted, he could hardly imagine their doing so.

That attitude, I am convinced, has kept count-
less men from obtaining the preventive screening
and early treatment that might have caught and
cured prostatic carcinoma before it killed them or
required treatment certain to produce the very
condition they most feared. Incredibly, laymen
are not alone in their reticence. In several books
and articles I read, the authors told of patients
whose physicians, including urologists, had not
explained that surgery or radiation might leave
them incontinent or impotent.

I subscribe to almost all the conventions of
polite conversation. Profanity is not one of my
vices, I don't tell dirty jokes, I seldom issue
reports on the state of my intestinal track, and
Patricia and I have never thought it appropriate to
tell our children at breakfast about the fine time
we had in the sack the night before. In that same
general spirit of discretion, I didn't talk to my students or second-circle friends about my own
apprehensions. On the other hand, talking with
close friends about prostate cancer without mentioning the possibility of incontinence or impotence seemed as shortsighted as talking about
Alzheimer's without mentioning memory loss or
of kidney failure with no discussion of transplants
or dialysis. Or, perhaps more fittingly, to discuss
breast cancer without considering the effects a mas-
tectomy might have on a woman's sense of self.

I could not predict just how the loss of urinary control or sexual potency might affect me. I was certain it would not enhance my self-image, but perhaps I would handle it reasonably well. Important as it was in my life, sexual activity did not involve large blocks of my time on a daily basis. Most of what gives meaning—family, friends, teaching, reading, writing, movies, bicycling, squash, skiing, good food—would still be there and there was little reason to think that my capacity for any of them, with the short-term exception of bicycling, would be diminished in any way. When it came to sex itself, I knew I could depend on Patricia's love and understanding and humor, and I was becoming increasingly open to the assistance of chemistry and bio-engineering. As I learned more about an apparently thriving industry dedicated to minimizing social embarrassment and facilitating sexual function, I came to understand that my situation was far from unique. Talking helped. In one conversation with a person I know well but had not seen in some time, I mentioned my reluctance to consider such options as penile injections. "Don't knock it," my friend said. "It has brought a lot of pleasure at our home."

Not all the proffered support was spiritual or emotional. One long-time friend called and revealed that he, too, had prostate cancer. He offered to share the fruits of his own explorations into alternative treatments. Not wishing to risk the side effects of either radiation or surgery, he was following a course of hormone therapy, which had significantly reduced his PSA count in a matter of less than six months. He was aware that suppression of a tumor by hormone therapy might be only temporary, but was willing to take a chance on it, while being careful to keep a close watch for any ominous signs—primarily a rise in his PSA count. If the tumor should resume its growth, he would consider cryosurgery, a new and less invasive technique in which probes filled with liquid nitrogen are inserted into the prostate to destroy it by freezing. The foremost practitioner of this technique, Dr. Gary Onik of the Allegheny General Hospital in Pittsburgh, confidently expects cryosurgery will be the technique of choice within a very few years, but it is still in the experimental stage and its results on the three key dimensions—survival and preservation of continence and potency—are not yet comparable to those for conventional surgery performed by experts. Because of growing satisfaction with surgical outcomes, urologists have not rushed to embrace the newer technique, tending to see it mainly as an alternative for patients who need a prostatectomy but for whom conventional surgery would pose an unacceptable risk.

My friend, who asked me not to tell others of his condition, loaned me a sizable stack of literature on alternative therapies and put me in touch with an organization known as PAACT (for Patient Advocates for Advanced Cancer Treatments), which also provided a substantial addition to my growing set of files. After reading these materials, which spoke not only of hormone therapy and crysosurgery, but also of preventions and treatment with vitamins and other substances, I concluded that they held promise and should be further investigated and developed. That, however, was a task for researchers and men who might get prostate cancer at some time in the future. For men like me, with a definitively diagnosed cancer of an apparently aggressive sort, and with access to a top-flight surgeon, the prostatectomy still seemed the appropriate route. I can't say with certainty how I would have reacted to this information if I had received it prior to deciding to have the surgery. I find it entirely plausible that, within ten years, treatment may exist that will make the nerve-sparing method of retropubic prostatectomy seem extreme or even clumsy, but these speculations were overcome by my gratitude that I had not been diagnosed with this disease in 1981, before Dr. Walsh's landmark achievements.

In my heart, I tend to believe the best. I recognize that most people who receive mailings informing them that they have definitely won a Mercedes-Benz, a Sony TV set, or a priceless piece of art will probably receive the art, which will be priceless for a good reason. Still, I have always felt I had a decent chance at the car or, at the least, a fine television set, and that sitting through a sales presentation regarding time-share resort properties would be a small price to pay for such a reward. (Patricia, fortunately, is more skeptical, and the requirement that I bring a registered spouse to such meetings has saved me from many wasted hours.) I also tend to feel that I have at least a reasonable chance to win the Reader's Digest Sweepstakes, especially after I learn that I have already passed through the first two stages and have been asked to specify what mode of travel I want to use when I go to Pleasantville to receive the first check. Why would they ask something like that if I were not on the short list?

Fortunately, this tendency, which I prefer to characterize as trusting rather than gullible, exists in tension with a non-risk-taking cognitive component of my personality. I don't gamble, not even to play the lottery—well, perhaps when it reaches $40 or $50 million, but I would donate a substantial portion of my winnings to charity. Although trusting in hormones to keep a tumor in check, or relying on an experimental mode of treatment might be a viable option for some, I never seriously considered altering the course I had chosen. I think I fully realized how comfortable I was with my decision when, one in evening in Wimberley while Patricia and I were scraping windows and cleaning floors, an episode of the syndicated television program, "The Crusaders," dealt with cancer clinics in Tijuana, focusing mainly on the exploitation of people desperate enough to pay large sums for dubious or decidedly fraudulent therapies. At one point, Patricia asked if it bothered me to listen to that program, and I realized that I had hardly made any connection to my own situation. I can't say what I would do if I were desperate, but as I had listened, I had been wondering how people could possibly fall for some of the more outrageous scams.

Two other good friends, Hank and Demaris, helped me add to my fund of knowledge by inviting us to a meeting of the Friends of Baylor College of Medicine at the River Oaks Country Club, at which Peter Scardino would speak about prostate cancer. Since my feelings toward Dr. Scardino were rapidly approaching reverence, I was grateful to have the opportunity to listen to him speak at length about my most pressing current interest. Speaking to an audience of several hundred affluent Houstonians, he talked first of the numerous accomplishments of Baylor's Department of Urology.

He spoke of the dissolution of kidney stones by means of shock waves, a technique that has virtually eliminated the need for surgery in treating calculi, and mentioned the development of prostheses for both incontinence and impotence. Then, he turned to the subject of prostate cancer.

He reported that the National Cancer Institute had recently chosen Baylor as one of two "Specialized Programs of Research Excellence" in prostate cancer and had been awarded a large three-year renewable grant. Because Baylor had received the highest ranking of 25 applicants, it was designated the Matsunaga-Conte Center for Prostate Cancer Research, after the late Senator Spark Matsunaga (D-Hawaii) and Representative Silvio Conte (R-Massachusetts), both of whom had died of prostate cancer. The other center to be funded, he revealed in a good-humored but obviously satisfied manner, was the urology department at Johns Hopkins. I subsequently learned that Drs. Walsh and Scardino are good friends who work together in numerous ventures but who also, as one might expect, keep a close eye on the other's latest accomplishments.

Scardino ran through the statistics that had by now become familiar to me, noting that three percent of men over 50 will die of prostate cancer and that something other than wider testing is making the disease increasingly common. He then turned to the controversy that surrounds prostate cancer and the choice of appropriate treatment. Pointing out that, in contrast to most forms of cancer, prostate cancer is slow-growing, he estimated that a prostatic carcinoma will double every two years and that it may take 25-30 years for the average tumor to become a killer. He stressed, however, that, though slow in its growth, it does not stop, a fact that makes it seem prudent to find it early and do something about it at that time. The average age of diagnosis, he said, is 70. The average of treatable diagnosis is 63, when a healthy man can expect to live an additional 18 years. He referred to an article in *The New York Times* which had asserted there is no way to tell a difference between a slow-growing and fast-growing tumor, and denied this is the case. He cited the familiar figure that one-third of men over 50 have cancer cells in their body, but strongly asserted that most of these are so microscopic as to make it dubious even to label them as cancer. The cells found in autopsy, he said, are 1/100th the size of the small tumors he and his colleagues are treating in the clinic. "They are," he said, "about as much alike as an acorn and an oak tree."

Scardino acknowledged that much remains to be learned about prostate cancer and that it would take 10-20 years of randomized testing, which is only now beginning, to have a firmer grasp on some of the crucial variables of the disease. He concluded that segment of his talk with a sentence that warmed my heart: "If we get a nasty cancer that is still in the capsule, we can almost always cure it."

He drew attention to a large national study to see if finasteride, the active ingredient in Merck's Proscar, could not only reduce BPH, but also prevent cancer, by lowering levels of DHT (dihydrotestosterone), the androgen most often suspected of promoting prostate cancer. He stressed that basic research is the only genuine hope for discovering a way to prevent the disease and noted that, because it is possible to start a prostate cancer from scratch in a mouse and go through a process in four weeks that would take 30 years in a man, scientists are coming closer to understanding what is going on, thus greatly facilitating both prevention and effective treatment. As for Proscar's ability to treat BPH, he observed that half the people in one controlled test had reported they had been helped by the drug. He added, however, that one-third of subjects who received a placebo reported it was the best thing they had ever tried.

Dr. Scardino mentioned that vitamin A-like drugs called retinoids can cause some cancer to reduce to a well-differentiated and less dangerous stage, and that this holds out promising hope for prevention and less aggressive forms of therapy. While he labeled the current enthusiasm for using vitamins to prevent cancer as "trendy," he acknowledged that "they probably play a role" and that their effectiveness should be investigated further. He also admitted he was intrigued by the possibility that zinc, often touted as "the male mineral," might truly prove useful in preventing BPH and prostate cancer, but said that studies had not yet shown sufficiently promising results.

He spoke of the importance of the PSA in early detection, giving figures that squared with what I had heard before. "Over 4, we worry. Over 10, we get quite worried. At the same time, some men can have a PSA count of 50 or even 80 and not have prostate cancer." He went on to note that the most valuable use of the PSA may be as a marker to see whether treatment has been successful. If the PSA rises after radiation or hormone therapy, one recognizes that the cancer is on the march again. If, after surgery, it does not fall to zero and remain there, it is clear that not all of the cancer, either at the site or elsewhere, was removed, and that adjuvant therapy may be called for.

I was curious to learn if Dr. Scardino had any opinion on cryosurgery, but since I had just signed on as his patient, it seemed imprudent to give the impression that I was having second thoughts. To my pleasure, one of the first persons to speak during the question session raised the topic. Scardino's answer struck me as cautious, but eminently fair. "I hope it will turn out to be an advance," he said, "but it's far too early to say. Excitement and hope might cloud reality. I suppose my position is why go for that when a proven treatment is available?"

In a parting shot, Dr. Scardino urged every man over 50, which included virtually every male in the room, to have a DRE and PSA test every year. "Waiting for symptoms to appear," he said, "is not the way to approach this disease."

Two days later, at my follow-up visit with the doctor, I told him I had been in the audience at the Friends of Baylor meeting and asked him to elaborate on a few matters, cryosurgery in particular. He explained that the crucial problem with cryosurgery is balancing safety and effectiveness. It is quite possible, he said, to be certain that radiation will completely destroy a prostatic cancer, but it might require burning a hole through a person's body. Cryosurgery has also resulted in some unnecessary damage to tissue. It had taken 25 years for radiologists to achieve an acceptable balance, he said, and he thought the chances were "pretty darn slim" that cryosurgery would prove to be safer and more effective than radiation.

In fairness, which seems to be a fine trait of his, Scardino noted that radiation is safer than surgery, though not as effective. He thought it reasonable to believe that at least 60 percent of men treated with radiation would have cancer cells present in biopsied tissue within two to four years; about 50 percent show a rise in their PSA count within five years. In contrast, he felt my chances of being completely clear at five years were at least 75 percent; if the cancer proved to be truly contained, the odds rose to nearly 95 percent, a figure I had heard him cite before, but did not resent hearing again. On a final positive note, he informed me that he had looked at my records and, because my tumor appeared to be at the base of the gland rather than the apex where the nerve bundles are located, the chances of saving both sets were good.

We settled on November 15, eleven days away, as the date for surgery, and he directed me to the ultrasound lab for another test, this one to check the state of my kidneys, to make sure they were healthy and also to determine whether some other kind of surgery might need to be performed while he was in there. To my satisfaction, this test did not require invasion of my body. The technician merely moved his lubricated ultrasonic wand along the bare skin in my kidney area. To my slight consternation, he and a urology resident sitting in on the session agreed that I had a cyst

about the size of a tennis ball on one of my kidneys. They showed it to me on the screen. Before
consternation could turn to alarm, they assured
me that such growths are not particularly uncommon, that urologists do not know what causes
them, and that they seldom cause any problems.
Dr. Scardino would probably not do anything
about it and, in time, it might go away. One good
thing about cancer is that it tends to make lesser
problems recede from consciousness. Disquieted
as I might have been, in normal times, to learn
that I have a tennis-ball sized foreign object
attached to one of my vital organs, I cannot recall
having thought about this matter even once until
sitting here four months later to write about it.

I could not be certain I was doing the right
thing, but I was satisfied I had made a good effort
to understand my disease, to consider the options
open to me, and to obtain first-rate care. I was
mostly at peace with my decision, and just about
over feeling sorry for myself. A dear friend, obviously filled with consternation, observed that
"Life is not fair," that my being struck with cancer
at this time in my life—with my career going well,
our children grown and happily married and producing offspring, and our long-awaited house in
the Hill Country finally finished—seemed incom-
prehensible. I cherished her loving bewilderment
but could not muster much sense of outrage. If

life were fair, I might not have discovered my tumor until it was too late. I might not have known how to negotiate the corridors leading to reliable information about the disease and its treatment. I might not have been able to afford or gain access to treatment as expert as any in the world. And, of course, I might not live in a web of love and friendship that seemed capable of holding me tightly, no matter how this all turned out.

I was in no mood to ask for justice.

CHAPTER 8

SURGERY

The last ten days before surgery passed swiftly. Predictably, I continued my reading about prostate cancer, taking special comfort in articles commending the surgical option, much as a new car owner enjoys reading positive stories about the brand and model he has just purchased. Dr. Scardino and the urology department's Senior Medical Editor, Carolyn Schum, a friend from another era whom I had not seen in years, helped by loading me down with the latest books and articles on the subject. They also urged me to contact Richard Howe, a former president of Pennzoil who underwent a successful prostatectomy in 1991 and has since devoted an enormous amount of time to promoting awareness of the disease and providing support to those who have it, and working closely with US TOO, the International Prostate Cancer Support Group. During several conversations, Dick gave me a detailed account of what I could expect in the hospital, things I needed to make sure the nurses attended to, and how soon I could expect to be back on my feet.

On the first weekend in November, Patricia and

I took John, our guest from Cambridge, to see the Alamo in San Antonio (his request) and then backtracked to Wimberley. The weather and the days were perfect—bright, cool, and bracing—and once again I ached at contemplating the possibility that I might not grow old in that sublime setting. In the evening we enjoyed the sunset from the porch and then walked quietly to the east side of the house to watch the herd of deer gather at twilight among the oak trees less than thirty yards away. The next day, we introduced John to Curlo and Margie, perfect neighbors who continue to teach us the secrets of country living, and Curlo told of spending time in Britain while waiting to sail to northern France, where he landed at Omaha Beach on D-Day.

Back in Houston, I tried to set my house in order. Chandler agreed to serve as acting chairman while I was away, and Angela agreed to teach two of my classes. I videotaped three other lectures, so that I had to cancel only two sessions before the semester ended, one of which was the Wednesday afternoon before Thanksgiving, when attendance is typically quite sparse. I signed papers stating that I would be on medical leave of absence for six weeks, and made sure I knew how to handle the insurance. I arranged to obtain a portable computer to see me through the recovery period, since I would not be able to sit at a regular desk for several weeks. And I caught up on the bills and went through stacks of mail and papers and magazines, in an effort to make room for the stacks that would arrive while I was incapacitated.

The perceptive reader may discern that I have a tendency toward workaholism. In newspaper tests that recommend therapy to those who place a check by as many as six of ten statements describing compulsive work habits, I seldom score less than eight and usually feel I could get a perfect score if I had thirty minutes to improve the test. As I filled several days with these mundane tasks, Patricia finally asked if I intended to work right up until she drove me to the hospital, or would I possibly consider going somewhere and spending a few days with her? As I have indicated, she takes the ending of eras seriously. Even if I recovered fully, we were facing a long dry spell and she clearly felt we needed to be banking some memories. She mentioned spending a few days at a luxury resort. We compromised by deciding to go back to Wimberley for one last pre-impotent weekend.

Sometime mid-week, Jeff called to say that, if we were agreeable, he and Samantha would like to meet us in Austin on Saturday, spend some time at Wimberley, visit Patricia's parents and several cousins in Austin for lunch on Sunday, and then fly back to L.A. in the afternoon. We were touched and delighted, but also aware that the last romantic weekend of 1993 would inevitably assume a different character than we had planned.

I was scheduled to check into the hospital by about 4:00 on Sunday afternoon, which meant I needed to leave Wimberley by noon. Jeff could rent a car in Austin, but to maximize time with them and also to give Patricia a chance to visit with her parents, we decided to take both cars. I would check in on my own and she could drop by the hospital in the evening. It meant both of us would spend several hours alone on the highway at a time when we would prefer to be together, but it seemed like the best solution.

We didn't get off as early as we had hoped to on Friday, and when we finally made it to the hilltop, we were both fairly tired. We watched the news to see what the weather would be and drank a glass of wine. We made love, sincerely but not spectacularly, and promised each other that Saturday night, children or no children, would be an affair to remember.

Jeff is an easy guest and we all took pleasure at watching Samantha pick up nails left by carpenters and marvel at the prickly pear and deer and cows and fire ants, none of which are indigenous to Brentwood, California. Saturday evening, we went to dinner at the Cypress Creek Cafe, where we ate the national dish of Texas, chicken-fried steak with mashed potatoes and cream gravy. (It may not be entirely risk-free, but patriotism requires sacrifice.) Back at the house, we fell naturally to talking about Jeff's career. Patricia and I were truly interested and the conversation continued longer than we had planned. We made it to the bedroom around midnight. Alone at last, we kissed, then lay back hesitantly. Finally, we laughed ruefully and admitted to each other that we were too tired to fulfill our promise. So it goes.

Sunday morning passed quickly and soon it was time to leave. Samantha hasn't been around us much, so it usually takes her some time to get past the awkwardness of fitting us into her emotional schema. I don't know what she knew about what I was facing, but when I stooped down to tell her good-bye and that I loved her, she hugged me warmly and said, "I love you, too, Granddad," in a tone that made me believe it. Jeff also gave me a big hug and said he would be in touch with Mom and Rex the next day. Patricia said she would see me in a few hours, and they drove off down the hill.

In the thirty-one days that had passed since Dr. Carlton had told me I had cancer, I had shed some tears, but I had never come close to losing control. I had not struggled with my composure, nor had I felt any strong need to keep up a good front. That's just the way it was. Now, to my utter surprise, as I walked back toward the house to lock up, I broke into racking sobs of an intensity greater than any I could ever remember. I knew enough about grieving to recognize that I may have been repressing something that needed to come out, so I decided to let it run for as long as it wanted to. Inside the house, I leaned on the couch, fully involved but also fascinated by what was going on. After about a minute, perhaps a little less, the storm cleared as suddenly as it had appeared. I washed my face, took another drink of apple juice (the only nourishment I was allowed all day other than clear broth), climbed into the pickup and drove to Houston, happily listening to the Oilers all the way.

Around 4:30 that afternoon, Rex came by to take me to the hospital. Though I felt fine and was traveling light, he insisted on carrying my bags. We checked in at the reception desk, which looked far more like that of a luxury hotel than of a hospital, then made our way to the urology ward on the fifth floor, which looked far more like a hospital than a luxury hotel. The first person to check on me after I settled into the room was an anesthesiologist whom Rex recognized as the brother of a friend of his from law school. After recalling when and where they had met, the doctor got down to business. As he looked at my chart, his eyes seemed teary, which caused me momentary anxiety, until he said, "You're fortunate to have caught this early. My father died of prostate cancer."

In my previous experiences at Methodist, I had been impressed with the thoroughness with which various procedures were explained and at the degree to which my own preferences were taken into account. The trend was holding. The doctor explained that, shortly before the operation I would receive a shot of Versed, a valium derivative that would calm me down and erase my memory of the entire pre-operative period. I told him I didn't suffer from excitability and that I saw little advantage in having my memory blotted out. Before two previous hand surgeries for old typing injuries, I had received what a nurse described as a "one-Margarita dose," which had relaxed me but enabled to me carry on conversation during the surgery and remember most of it when it was over. I didn't expect to remain conscious during this operation, but I would prefer to concentrate more on killing pain than blotting out memories. "That's fine," he said. "We'll cut back the dose. It won't effect the pain of the surgery at all. It's just to calm you down. Some people get pretty anxious. When Jerry Lewis was in here, he was bouncing off the walls." Well, Jerry and I often react differently to things.

After my medical Margarita, I would be wheeled to the preparation room and an epidural catheter would be inserted into my back, next to the spinal cord. This would be the primary conduit of the painkillers I would receive, applying them at the point of greatest need rather than flooding my entire system with drugs. He touted this as a great innovation in pain management that would not only eliminate most of the pain formerly associated with this operation, but would do so without making me feel too dopey. It would remain in place for several days and I would be able to punch a button and administer a dose of painkiller whenever I needed it. During the operation itself, I would also be given a general anesthetic, first through an IV and then through a tube in my throat. I could expect to feel some soreness in my throat afterward, but this would quickly pass.

My hand surgeries had all been scheduled for the early morning, and I knew that Dr. Scardino was usually through by noon. I was surprised, then, when the anesthesiologist told me they would come get me about 11:00 A.M. and that the operation would start about noon. "You're his second patient of the day," he explained. So that was how I managed to get on his schedule.

"Will that be a problem?" I asked, not wanting my surgeon to be at less than his best.

"Not at all. The first one will just be batting practice. When he gets to you, he'll be all warmed up."

A comforting image. I thought about it for a moment and decided there was no point in finding anything new to worry about.

Rex went home shortly after the anesthesiologist left, and I found myself, like Charlie Chaplin in that famous picture, caught up in the gears of a quite large and efficient machine. First came a "clear dinner," consisting entirely of water in several forms: Jello, pineapple juice, fruit ice, and tea. Then came a steady stream of technicians, nurses, and administrators. Aaron rearranged some items in the room and asked me how many pillows I thought I would need, recommending that I order an extra just to hold against my stitches when I coughed, to fight the pain. That proved to be an excellent suggestion. Nick brought a plastic device with a breathing tube attached and showed me how to raise and suspend a little plastic float for a second or two by inhaling and holding my breath. He said I would find it a difficult feat after the surgery, but must remember to attempt it every hour or two whenever I was awake.

Another technician arrived with a wheelchair and said he needed to take me to the X-ray lab. He seemed surprised when I told him I could walk. "Are you sure? It's on the third floor." I assured him I could handle it. "I'm not sick," I explained. "I just have cancer. I feel fine. Come back tomorrow when I'm cured. That's when I'll need your chair." In the lab, I sat next to a man who was clearly sick, and I realized once again what a blessing it had been to have lived my first 55 years in good health, and wondered if this would be the last day on which I would be able to think of myself as a healthy person.

Patricia was waiting in the room when I returned from the X-ray lab, and she reported on her visit with her family. Since I was scheduled for midday, which meant she could easily see me the next morning, she decided to go home and let the staff members continue their work.

Aaron reappeared to give me a pill that would stimulate my stomach to empty and administered a Fleet enema that took care of the job the rest of the way down. Nurse Bacero explained that, before I would be ready to go home, my now-empty and idle intestines would need to revive, which could be slow to occur. "The guts," she said, "are the last people to wake up after an operation."

An administrator gave me a sheaf of materials to read and forms to sign, giving permission to perform various procedures and stipulating that I understood the various risks involved and would not hold Methodist Hospital responsible for unavoidable bad results. I did not find it comforting to be reminded of what I might be surrendering on the morrow, but I signed. After she left, I read through the materials one last time and noticed that I had authorized Dr. Scardino to perform any procedure he deemed necessary after he got inside. I wondered if that included an orchiectomy. I hoped not. I did not want my orchids clipped without further discussion with the gardener.

One form that had somehow escaped my attention offered me the opportunity to donate any organs I no longer planned to use. I believe in organ donation, but I didn't think there would be much demand for a used prostate, and I was reluctant to make anything else available at just this time. Perhaps I would sign that one when I didn't feel quite so vulnerable.

Interestingly, I had gained so much confidence in Peter Scardino and the nerve-sparing surgical technique that I had come to feel reasonably secure about my chances of regaining urinary control and potency. Now, with less than 24 hours to go, I began to worry once again about survival. To be sure, a one-in-twenty chance of lymph-node involvement justified optimism, but it was not a sure thing. My last visitor of the evening helped put my mind at ease. A urology resident came in for a final check, to see if I had any questions. He didn't seem in a hurry and we had a good conversation. He noted that, at my age and general condition, I could expect to rebound from the operation rather quickly. I told him I wasn't really worried about recuperating from the surgery. I just hoped I had some serious surgery to recuperate from, because that would mean my lymph nodes were clear and Dr. Scardino had in fact removed my prostate.

Dick Howe had told me that when he woke up in the recovery room, it took him twenty minutes to find someone who could tell him whether his prostate had been removed, and that this had caused him considerable agitation. He had given me a simple tip that, if I could remember it, would spare me this problem. All I had to do was reach down and feel my penis. If it had a catheter running through it, the operation had been completed. I shared that bit of intelligence with the resident. He smiled but said that would not be necessary. "Your prostate is coming out. I'm 99 percent sure of that. I've been on this service for 8 months and I haven't seen a single person with your numbers who's had lymph-node involvement. You're going to be fine." I decided to believe him. Within a few minutes, I went to sleep and, with the exception of the last two prostate-related episodes of nocturia I would ever experience, slept well until morning.

I would have preferred to have been waked up, wheeled down the hall, and operated on, with minimal time for reflection, but it wasn't my call. Patricia came to my room and we read the paper and talked a bit, but I don't remember any heavy-duty, last-minute expressions of fear or anxiety. This was what we had chosen and we were ready to get on with it. The operation in front of mine took about an hour longer than expected but, soon enough, they came to get me. Patricia and I kissed, with a recognition that this was momentous, but also with the full expectation that we would be seeing each other again in just a few hours.

I had requested that Dr. Alex Rosas serve as anesthesiologist on the surgery and was pleased when Dr. Scardino pronounced that an excellent choice. Dr. Rosas is married to Patricia's gynecologist and has an excellent reputation. In addition, we had met socially and had learned that he and his wife enjoy bicycling in the Wimberley area, so I figured we would get to know both of them better in the future. If I have to surrender control of my body to someone else, I prefer it be someone I know and like.

The first order of business after we got to the preparation room was to place the epidural catheter in my back. With the aid of a shot of xylocaine, it was a painless procedure and I was

pleased to have Dr. Rosas second his colleague's
opinion that this relatively recent tool has been
one of the greatest improvements in the management of post-surgical pain. He recommended that
I not make any major business deals or assume
that any sentences I happened to write were as
brilliant as they might seem at the moment, but
promised I would feel less pain and less woozi-
ness than with earlier forms of anesthetics.

A nurse shaved my stomach. Later in the
process, after I went under, someone completed
the process on the rest of the surgical region in a
manner so thorough as to make me wonder just
how it was done.

At last, it was time. As I was rolled into place,
Dr. Rosas told me that this was the operating
room used by Dr. Michael DeBakey, the legendary
Baylor/Methodist surgeon who pioneered and
perfected many of the techniques of open-heart
surgery. Looking up, I could see the windows
through which observers had viewed those his-
toric operations. And then I was gone.

I remember nothing else, but from watching a
video of the operation—not my own, but that of
some prostatic Everyman—I know approximately
what happened. After making a vertical incision
of about eight inches, from the navel to the pubic
bone, the first order of business was to remove the
lymph nodes and send them upstairs to see if they

contained evidence of cancer. I had imagined the lymph nodes were about the size of a lima bean, but they appeared to be about the size of an egg. I could not help wondering if they weren't something I would miss. (In fact, they are bean-sized. What I saw were the egg-sized pads of fat that surround them.)

The instant pathology exam took about twenty minutes. Patricia is not the sort to have wanted a roomful of friends and relatives hovering around her for hours in the waiting room. On the other hand, she didn't want to be alone in case the report on the nodes was a bad one. Rex, the natural and best choice to wait with her, was there, as both of us knew he would be. To her surprise, Fred, a friend from Austin, showed up as well. But then, no one who knows Fred is ever truly surprised at his generosity of spirit toward his friends. He knew the stages of my operation and had driven 180 miles to be with Patricia until she got the news about the nodes. As soon as Dr. Scardino's associate came out to report that the nodes were clear and the operation would proceed, he told Rex and Patricia good-bye and headed back to Austin. Several years ago, doctors discovered a tumor near the front of Fred's brain. He and his wife Kathy invited us to spend a few days with them at South Padre Island over the weekend before he was to undergo exploratory surgery.

We agreed; then, because of pressing commit-
ments, we backed out. Fred wouldn't have done
that. Fortunately, his tumor was just a knot, and
he is still around to give lessons in friendship.

In the two hours that followed, Dr. Scardino
clamped and tied off veins in the pelvic region,
enabling him to see what was he was doing. He
then inserted a Foley catheter through the urethra
and into the bladder. The Foley catheter is an
ingenious device; made of heavy-duty silicone,
the part that goes into the bladder is encased in a
small balloon which is inflated with water once it
is inside the bladder. This keeps it from slipping
out. As the operation progressed, Dr. Scardino
used it as a lever to move the prostate into position for the various cuts—all, to my surprise,
made with scissors rather than a scalpel. With
painstaking care, he identified the nerve bundles
and separated them from the gland, then set the
prostate free, snipping the urethra at the neck of
the bladder and again just below the prostate,
which enabled him to remove the troublesome
member from my body, hanging on the catheter
like a hideous bead on a string. After the bladder
neck and the urethral stump were properly prepared, a new catheter was inserted and inflated. I
never saw the first one; I would get to know this
one well. With the catheter serving as an internal
splint, the bladder neck was drawn down to the

urethral stump and the connection, known as an anastamosis, was made. After reattaching various blood vessels and inserting drains that would draw off blood and other fluids over the next few days, my remaining parts were put back into place as neatly as possible and the incision was closed.

I was, of course, quite unaware of all this. I had expected to struggle out of a deep fog and had wondered how long it would take, after I began to regain consciousness, to realize where I was and to start trying to find out precisely which of the possible outcomes had been attained. I do not know if the sparing use of general anesthetic made my return to wakefulness easy. All I know, all I care about knowing, is that the first words I heard, from a green-clad medical person I did not recognize—were entirely comprehensible and wonderfully welcome: "The lymph nodes were clear, and we spared both nerve bundles."

"What about blood," I asked.

"You didn't need any."

I raised clenched fists in grateful triumph. Three for three.

CHAPTER 9

RECOVERY

Soon after I woke up, I was wheeled back to my room, where Patricia was waiting. She reported what Dr. Scardino had told her after the operation. As best he could tell by visual and tactile examination, my tumor had been about the size of a finger joint—much bigger than a BB. Unlike approximately 90 percent of prostatic tumors, it had been located in the center of the gland, which helped account for the severity of my urinary difficulties and explained why neither DRE nor TRUS had picked it up. Fortunately, it also meant that it was less likely to have penetrated the capsule. We wouldn't know about that with certainty until early January, when the pathology report would be complete, but the signs were excellent. In all likelihood, I had been cured of prostate cancer.

With that news in hand and all pain still in abeyance, we began to examine the patient. First, of course, was my scar. Richard "Racehorse" Haynes, a colorful Houston criminal lawyer, tells of having questioned a woman who had been shot by the wife of a jealous husband. When he asked her to confirm that she had been "shot in the fracas," she replied, "Actually, it was between the navel and the fracas." Well, I had a neatly sewn scar running the full distance between my navel and my "fracas." A nurse commented that it looked good enough to have been done by a plastic surgeon, and I began to feel quite proud of it.

Next, we checked out the catheter. On first glance, I wondered if Dr. Scardino had failed to give Patricia a full report. My genitals, responding to both the trauma and blood loss, had shrunk and receded into my body to such an extent that they would surely have been safe from Lorena Bobbitt. Close inspection, however, reassured me that all the vital parts were there. It also revealed the catheter tube that would drain my bladder continually, minimizing leakage of urine into the repair site until the bond between the bladder neck and urethral stump became watertight. The tube was thicker in diameter than I had expected, but there seemed to be room for it, and a check of the bag hanging on the edge of the bed confirmed that it was doing its job.

I had fully expected the scar, the catheter, the epidural pain-management tube, and assorted IVs, but three other items surprised me. On each side of the scar, about four inches south of my navel and three inches east and west, was a Jackson-Pratt drain. These comprised a flexible plastic tube running from the operation site, through a snug-fitting (but not sutured) hole in my skin, to gathering devices that resembled clear hand grenades. When first attached, the grenades were squeezed, creating a suction that kept blood, urine, and other liquids from collecting in the pelvic region. When full, the collecting bottle would be emptied, squeezed again, and reattached to the tube.

One needed only to look at the two bloody grenades to discern what they did and to see that they worked. The third item posed a greater challenge. On the right side, midway between the scar line and the drain, a little coil of thick plastic thread was Scotch-taped to my stomach. One end entered my body as if run through my skin with a large needle; the other end was attached to an ordinary button. I entertained several hypotheses. Perhaps, by attaching a Dixie Cup to the button, I would be able to receive bulletins from a little biodegradable homunculus left inside to send dispatches from the front. Or perhaps it would be used, like a lawnmower cord, to jump-start my nerve bundles in case normal recovery occurred too slowly. The correct explanation was less fanciful, but hardly the sort of thing one associates with high-tech medicine. The other end of the string ran through the wall of my bladder and was tied to an eye, like that of a large needle, in the tip of the Foley catheter just above the balloon.

If the balloon unexpectedly deflated and the catheter slipped out, the string could be used to hoist a new one into place. The button was simply to keep the string from slipping back into the abdominal cavity.

My final new appendages had been explained to me, but I had not yet seen them in action. These constituted a Sequential Compression Device designed to prevent blood clots from forming in my legs while I as bedridden. My legs, in elastic stockings, were encased in plastic coverings outfitted with inflatable panels, like a child-sized swimming-pool raft. An air compressor huffing away under the bed filled these air-pockets sequentially, from the ankles upward, then relaxed and repeated the cycle, making sure my blood was never able to hang around in some joint and form a conspiracy against me. If the leggings got too warm, a flick of a switch would send cool air hissing through dozens of small holes.

As one can imagine, I felt helpless and entirely dependent upon the kindness of strangers, but I also felt an overwhelming sense of relief, joy, and gratitude. All things considered, this had been a fine day.

When Patricia left for the night, I tried to sleep but had difficulty, probably because I'd had a five-hour nap that afternoon. I was neither edgy nor in pain, and spent much of the night planning my course for the spring semester. Cancer cured; back to work.

On Tuesday morning, David Bybee came to see me during his rounds. When he asked how I felt, I told him that the only time it hurt was when I got an erection. He said, "That's almost a sick joke," but he was genuinely tickled, which pleased me.

A little while later, Dr. Scardino came in for a quick visit before departing for Sicily. He repeated what he had told Patricia, adding that, although the nerve bundles had been arranged more tightly along the edge of my prostate than he hoped, he felt he not had to damage even a single nerve. "I don't know how it could have gone any better," he said. Sometimes that's the way things happen in an unfair world.

The rest of the day went reasonably well. I had a dozen or so visitors and I talked on the phone to others. I was still giddy with relief, but by the end of the day the joys of hospital life were fading and my system was beginning to rebel against the insult it had suffered. I was not allowed to eat or drink anything, but the constant trickle from the IV bag kept me from getting hungry or thirsty. It did not keep my mouth from getting dry, so I was permitted to suck on a small cup of ice every four or five hours and, as a special treat, to rub my gums and tongue with a lemon-glicerine swab.

When I sat up, I invariably became nauseated, but since I had nothing to lose, it resulted in a dry heave that produced a notable strain on my stitches, causing me to clutch desperately to the extra pillow Aaron had recommended I order. Bad as it felt, this was garden-variety nausea that usually passed quickly, but I thought of cancer patients who undergo an extended regimen of chemotherapy and wondered if the nausea that often accompanies it is not worse than pain.

The nausea, I learned, was a side effect of the pain medicine, as were chronic hyperacidity, a low-grade headache, and near-constant hiccups. Alteration of the analgesic mix reduced the acidity and headache. The hiccups, I was told, could be cured with thorazine, a remedy I declined from fear it might make me a less interesting person.

By late Tuesday evening, I was exhausted. To ease the passage from wakefulness, I reached for a crossword puzzle book I had brought with me. After a few minutes in the world of aretes, ediles, Otoes, and long-dead movie stars—a characteristic that suggests a strong correlation between the ages of crossword enthusiasts and prostate-cancer victims—I slipped into unconsciousness and slept a solid six hours without changing position.

Wednesday was harder and Thursday marked the nadir of my stay. The nausea and hiccups continued, and lying in one position, knees flexed

and back tilted upward to avoid straining the
stitches, grew increasingly onerous. Not until
midnight Wednesday did a nurse named Bob help
me find an alternate position, which gave me
some relief. All the nurses were cordial and com-
petent, but seriously overworked. Because a
number of patients had scheduled surgery with
an eye toward a pre-Christmas recovery and a
1993 tax deduction, the urology ward was packed.
Unfortunately, this coincided with a recent cost-
trimming cutback in the number of nurses per
shift. On several occasions when I truly needed a
nurse, the response was slow and accompanied by
frustrated apology. Repeatedly, when I was being
attended to, my nurses would receive calls to
come to other rooms, which meant they would
also arrive late and apologetically at the next
patient's room. To complicate matters further, the
entire ward was scheduled to be shifted to another floor on Saturday, and preparations for the
move added to an already frenetic atmosphere.

On Thursday, I took the first difficult steps of
my post-prostate era, with a nurse holding onto
one arm and the other steadied by a bent and rick-
ety IV/catheter pole—an ironic symbol of my current state, I thought. If the "Prime Time Live"
crew had visited this ward, I doubt Sam
Donaldson would have criticized Methodist
Hospital for its luxury-hotel atmosphere. My last

two visits to this institution had been to the ortho-
pedic surgery unit, from which most patients
walked out smiling a few hours after their operations, and to the maternity ward, with its warm
and joyful affirmation of new life. In stark contrast, the urology ward is filled with old men in
pain, depressed by their impotence, evidence of
their incontinence hanging in full view, and their
naked butts and hairless legs sticking out of back-
less hospital gowns. These, I thought, are "the
few, the humiliated, the Urine Corps." One look
at my new peer group moved me to suggest that it
might be best if would-be visitors just sent a note
or called. Men look better in our power suits.

As Nurse Bacero had warned me, the guts are
the last people to wake up after an operation, but
they would have to wake up before I would be
ready to go home, and that meant they would
have to have something to work with. On
Thursday, I began to receive food trays. What I
got seldom matched what I had checked on the
order form, but they were all items from the
restricted menu, and since no one form of water
seemed much more promising than any of the
others, that didn't bother me. On Thursday
evening, after a walk down Hell's Alley, I ingested
another of the chef's "clear" dinners, and sat in a
chair from the beginning of network news to the
end of McNeil-Lehrer. When I got up, I discov-

ered that the epidural catheter had come out. I was scheduled to keep it a day longer, but the pain-management technician decided to switch me to Percoset, a synthetic opiate. I wondered if losing my magic morphine machine meant I would have a rough night, but the technician assured me I could order a shot of Demerol or morphine any time I needed it. "There is nothing heroic about enduring pain," she said. "These drugs are made for precisely this purpose. Ask for them if you need them and don't worry about how much you should take. It's your body. What is normal for you is normal." In fact, the Percoset was quite adequate and removing the needle from my back meant I had one less tube to consider when I needed to move.

By Friday, I felt I had turned the corner, but the teams of residents and technicians who visited me each day sought tangible evidence that my gas-trointestinal track was back on the job. Specifically, they wanted a good-faith show of flatulence. I had quickly grown accustomed to having uniformed nurses give me sponge baths and change the dressing at the point where the catheter tube exited the head of my penis. I never did get used to having a perky young woman in street clothes ask if I had managed to pass any gas yet. The last time anyone had actually encour-aged me to fart had been on a Boy Scout camporee and, if I remember correctly, matches were involved. (For any women who may be reading this, it's a guy kind of thing.) I regarded their interest as bordering on the surreal, but when I finally managed to sing the song of the nether larynx, though it was hardly enough to hold back on an elevator, their joy was unmistakable. One auditor actually used the phrase, "music to our ears." Small victories.

As another sign of my recovery, my Jackson-Pratt drains, which had been running on empty, were removed. Dick Howe had told me this had been one of the most excruciatingly unpleasant aspects of his entire hospital stay, recalling that "I felt like my intestines were being pulled out." When I mentioned this to a nurse, she said most men compared it to sticking their finger in a light socket. Neither image was comforting. In my case, the reality turned out to be more agreeable. The resident who removed them, the first on Friday and the second on Saturday, asked me to take a deep breath and hold it, then quickly extracted the tube, closing the hole with a piece of tape. The momentary discomfort was no worse than one might feel if a piece of adhesive tape were pulled off a hairy leg, a small price to pay to be free of these man-made leeches.

On Friday evening, I read part of an Armistead Maupin novel and watched the David Letterman show before falling asleep. I knew I was getting well when I dreamt I had lost the notes for a speech I was supposed to give.

On Saturday, moving day, the hospital felt and sounded like a zoo under construction, causing me to be grateful the transfer had not occurred on Wednesday or Thursday, when I had felt so much worse. But the room was newly painted, with better lighting, and I was feeling stronger by the hour. I visited happily with Patricia and several friends who dropped in, and, finally, ate two real meals. For the better part of the afternoon, I sat in a chair—slanted back on my tailbone with a pillow under me and my feet propped up on an ottoman, but sitting nonetheless—and watched Boston College squeak out a victory over Notre Dame.

On Sunday, nurses checked me out on the controls of my catheter bag, making sure I knew how to switch from the large bedside bag I had worn all week to a smaller portable unit I could attach to my leg during the day, to facilitate mobility. I also received instruction regarding the array of medication being sent home with me: pain medicine (for which, happily, I had little need), laxatives and stool softeners to keep me from ripping stitches, iron pills to build up my red blood count, antibiotics to fend off infection, and salve to use when I changed my catheter dressing. And then, flowers proceeding on a cart in front of me and balloons flying from my wheelchair arm, we headed into the bright fall afternoon and home.

After getting settled into the bedroom, I took a short nap. When I awoke, our daughter Dale, who had volunteered to take care of me for a week while Patricia was at work, had arrived from Baton Rouge with baby Laura. Mary and Molly had also come over. The six of us, including Patricia, were sitting on our bed talking when the revivification of my intestines, so earnestly expected in the hospital, began to occur right before our ears. Stomachs merely growl. My pipes and tubes and hoses, from a point so high in my chest that I cannot imagine what was going on, to a location quite near the lower terminus, began to rumble and sputter like a hydraulic energy plant being put back into operation after years of sitting idle. For a minute or two, we all practiced what sociologists call "studied non-observance," but when I finally asked if I might be left alone for a few minutes, they scattered without a question. Alone at last, I achieved what may fairly be called a symphonic expression of systemic renewal.

Just before dinner, I went for a short walk in the cool twilight, in part to test my portable catheter bag, in part just to get outside. I quickly decided that, in man, PVC plumbing is a poor substitute for the real thing, and friction on the tubing limited my mobility. Still, as I shuffled along the leaf-

covered sidewalk, savoring the aroma drifting
from my neighbors' fireplaces and noticing how
magnificent an ordinary house on an ordinary
street could seem, I felt flooded with warm feelings toward my family, my neighbors, fall, smoke,
leaves, concrete—you name it, I loved it. I was
pleased my lease had been renewed.

My recovery went smoothly. I read and
watched one or two movies a day. With the
portable computer, I was able to keep up with cor-
respondence, prepare a final exam for my course,
and continue my lifelong habit of compulsive
note-taking. I couldn't sit upright, but by putting
most of my weight on my coccyx and keeping my
feet propped up, I was able to approximate a sitting position without much discomfort. I couldn't
drive or lift anything that weighed more than ten
pounds, both measures designed to keep me from
ripping a stitch. On the few occasions when I lift-
ed something close to the limit, I understood the
wisdom of this instruction. My energy level
seemed as high as it had been prior to the surgery,
proportionate to the tasks I had to perform.

My daily schedule, or lack of it, required so little of me that I often had trouble going to sleep at
the appropriate time. Several evenings I got up
and read—I have never learned to watch television in the middle of the night. One morning

about four, I had finished reading Donald Hall's *Life Work*, which begins by talking about work, but ends by talking about the cancer that developed while the book was in progress. *The New York Times* lands in my front yard quite early in the morning, and I thought it possible that it might already have arrived, so I decided to check. Since it comes wrapped in a blue plastic sleeve, it is difficult to spot in the dark, so I poked around here and there, trying in vain to locate it. After a few minutes, I gave up, my retreat into the house hastened by a pair of headlights heading in my direction. I had every right to be there, but I didn't want the constable or a neighbor to be alarmed at the sight of a gimpy old guy in striped shorts and baggy T-shirt standing in his yard holding a rope with a bag of pee on the end of it.

The catheter bag strapped to my leg proved to be an annoyance, but no more than that. On one occasion, it gave me momentary social cachet. David Berg and his fiancée, Kathryn, took us to breakfast one morning, and when we stopped by his house for a few minutes afterward, both their cats came and nuzzled up against my leg. Kathryn was impressed, noting that the cats usually did not like strangers. After noticing the precise focus of their interest, I suggested that they might be more attracted by my catheter spore than by any natural affinity for animals they might have sensed in me. David cackled with delight and, adopting the voice and role of a cat confiding in a companion, said, "He's tall, but I like him. Whaddya think?"

As I have mentioned, the sick role doesn't get one much in our family. On my second night home, I commented on how delicious Patricia's chicken and dumplings were. She replied, as sweetly as one can imagine, "I'm so glad you like them, Darling. Why don't you get yourself some more?"

Pat Meyers had warned that I should count on making no more than one or two trips between floors a day. I was free to do more, but she doubted I would feel like it. In fact, I found that, if I took it slowly, I had little difficulty negotiating stairs. I was also able to shower normally and eat anything I wished, as long as it was not constipating. Residents and nurses had told me to expect some swelling of my scrotum, probably to the size of a softball. Fortunately, I escaped that particular side effect altogether.

My homebound recovery period had no real low spots. Dale and I are soul mates and I cherished the chance to talk with her and get to know Laura better. But the unquestioned high point came on Wednesday morning, nine days after my operation. I awoke to an unfamiliar discomfort in the region of my catheter, which I taped to my leg at an angle to minimize irritating friction when I moved about. I reached a hand down, trying to figure out what was wrong, and then, I understood. I poked Patricia, gently but insistently, and spoke her name several times. When awakened instead of easing into consciousness on her own, she often responds with mild alarm. "What is it, Bill? Is something wrong? Is it your catheter? What can I do?"

"It's OK," I assured her. "Give me your hand."

In a moment, she confirmed my discovery. At 6:41 A.M. on November 24, 1993, nine days after surgery that might have left me impotent, we had concrete—well, not concrete, but reassuringly firm—evidence that we had been spared a traumatic loss. "Oh, Sweetheart!" she said. "I can't believe it." Since there was no obviously fitting way to celebrate, we just lay there on our backs, holding hands and giggling, while tears of relief rolled down our cheeks, and I thought of the first morning of our honeymoon, nearly 36 years earlier, when just hours into our status as former virgins, we lay beside each other in the Sun Valley Motel, looking forward with wonder to pleasures of the flesh that for so long had seemed unattainable. God bless you, St. Patrick and St. Peter, and thanks be given for the resurrection of the body. The next morning, at 5:24, according to my Sony Dream Machine, the phenomenon reappeared with even greater vigor, countering any lingering skepticism. It was Thanksgiving morning.

I was scheduled to have my catheter removed three weeks from the date of the surgery. Although it had not been painful, it was both a physical and logistical irritant and I looked forward ardently to emancipation day. I had been instructed to bring a couple of adult diapers with me, so Patricia and I went out one evening to the drug store. She tickled me by threatening to ask where she could find Huggie Supremes in the 190 to 210 pound size, but after we settled on some Depend Easy Fit adult diapers, with adjustable strap tabs by Velcro USA, she offered to take them to the counter as if they were hers, not mine. A touching gesture, I thought, but they were my diapers and I would carry them. Let the clerk think whatever she wanted to.

Pat Meyers handled the catheter removal on her own. First, she funneled a substantial amount of water through the catheter end of my bladder to establish that the network was secure and the urethra open. My bladder had never been filled from that end before and did not respond gracefully, choosing instead to expel most of the water immediately, which meant I would have to fill it in the normal way—from above, by drinking. Carefully explaining what she was going to do at every point, Pat then clipped the button and safety cord still taped outside my abdomen and slowly pulled the catheter out. The sensation was unique but not painful, and I was free at last, free at last. I slipped into one of my diapers, pulled on my trousers, and listened to her instructions and advice regarding my hoped-for return to continence and other aspects of my recuperation. Before long, my kidneys had processed enough liquid to give my new urethral path a fair test. I stepped into a rest room and discovered, as I had expected, that it all worked just fine. I was pleased, though not wholly surprised, to learn that I was able to halt the flow in mid-stream, a sign that eventual continence was virtually assured. To heighten my pleasure, I noted that my stream was more forceful and full than it had been in at least a decade.

I had joked that my three younger granddaughters and I could exchange notes with each other in 1994, as we all attacked the problem of toilet training. I had been warned not to expect anything in particular. Some men achieve satisfactory urinary control in a matter of two or three weeks. Most take three to six months, and some require a year or more. I take no personal credit and can offer no advice as to how one might obtain the same results, but I was one of the lucky ones. After two or three days with the big diapers, I was fairly certain they represented overkill. The absorbent male pouches advertised in the literature Pat Meyers gave me seemed too expensive, so I decided to experiment with something more cost-effective. I scored on the first try, when I discovered that one Kotex Maxipad slipped into a pair of jockey shorts gave me adequate protection for an entire day, though I usually carried a spare in the inside ticket pocket of my suit or blazer.

Over the two-week Christmas holiday, which we spent at Wimberley, where accidents were not likely to be detected, I graduated to a simple Lightdays Comfort-Design Pantiliner (unscented). After a few weeks at that stage, I decided to "go bare," as it were, with only occasional minor leakage. As I had been warned, caffeine, carbonated water, and alcohol all truly did pose a challenge, providing me with yet another impetus to healthy living.

Urination wasn't something I talked about much, but I admit to being pleased when a close friend would ask for specific details of my progress. And I experienced a real rush of satisfaction when, one day in a library rest room, I stood shoulder to shoulder with a man about my age, and while he waited and wiggled and grumbled and shook, I whooshed noisily, washed quickly, and whisked out of the room, hardly able to restrain myself from asking, "What did you think of that, Buster?"

We had a family gathering on Christmas Day,

and on New Year's Eve, my 56th birthday and our 36th anniversary—if you're doing the math, we waited so Patricia wouldn't have to marry a teenager—we were joined by Richard and Michael (his wife, not his special friend), with whom we have shared that happy occasion many times in the past. The rest of the time, it was just the two of us, which was what we wanted and cherished. Romance did not exactly bloom, but it budded enough to bring great pleasure and to provide definitive justification for our optimism.

As the idyll drew to a close, we acknowledged to each other a slight uneasiness about the pathology report we would receive a day after returning to Houston. Six weeks had passed since the operation. A pathology report can be done more quickly than that, but a combination of the holidays and the fact that my report would be passed around to interested parties within the Baylor clinic accounted for the delay. I did not expect bad news. If the examination had uncovered evidence of cancer cells in the surgical margins, surely I would have heard by now and been urged to begin additional therapy.

The news was indeed good, but not quite what we had expected. Dr. Scardino began by giving us the bottom line: There was no evidence of microscopic cancer cells in the surgical margins; therefore, no further treatment was indicated, and I should not have to worry about recurrence. Still, both Patricia and I noticed that he seemed subdued. "That," he said, referring to the tumor, "was a bad actor. It was two-and-a-half centimeters across at the greatest dimension, and it reached nearly all the way from the apex to the base. It had gotten into, but not through, the second layer [of "rind"]. If you had waited another year, I think it would have escaped." As supporting evidence, in the three months between my last visit with David Bybee and the surgery, my PSA had risen from 8.0 to just over 10.

We talked about how I was doing, and he registered his pleasure at my progress. He told me what kinds of improvements I could still anticipate and was pleased that I had begun writing about the experience. Patricia and I thanked him for his contribution to our lives, told him good-bye, and returned to work, but about mid-afternoon we talked on the telephone and admitted to each other that we had not found it easy to concentrate. We kept hearing, "If you had waited another year..." I had thought of having a bullet whiz by my head and lodge in a post; her image was seeing a bad car wreck in the rearview mirror just after passing through an intersection. Both of us had been reminded that our first fears were not groundless.

I think it possible that, in some cases, particularly courageous and strong-willed individuals may legitimately claim to have "beaten the Big C," to have struggled with a killer, undergone devastating therapy, and emerged victorious. I am not one of those heroic individuals. I discovered I had something that didn't hurt, looked carefully at the options, chose one that worked, and—as far as I can tell—got well. But the real credit for this victory goes to medical expertise, for whose value I have new and grateful regard. I am quite aware that many other men will not be so fortunate, but I sincerely hope that new attention to this disease will enable multitudes to find a resolution as satisfactory as mine has been. And I hope that physicians such as Patrick Walsh and Peter Scardino and their colleagues will find ways to prevent this disease and less traumatic ways to treat it.

In the time, still brief, that has passed, I have gone back to work with no discernible diminution of energy. I spend most of my days doing the same things I did before I learned I had cancer. But I am not the same. I take vitamins, I bought and use a juicer, I eat more grains and fresh fruits and vegetables than ever, and I attend US TOO support group meetings. But that is not what I am referring to. Almost every day, and often several times a day, I find myself taking conscious pleasure in some sight or sound or touch or taste that would have gone unnoticed before. I am increasingly able to distinguish between things I

could do and things I want and need to do,
between invitations I could accept and invitations
I want to accept. I am more self-conscious, but I
don't think I have become more selfish. In
response to the love and kindness and thoughtful-
ness so many expressed to me, I believe I am more
sensitive to the pain and vulnerabilities of others,
and more pleased and encouraging at their pleasures and triumphs. I am not a perfect husband
or father or grandfather, or an ideal teacher or colleague or neighbor or friend, and never will I be,
but I no longer imagine I have limitless time to
meet unrealistic expectations, so I make my lists of
who and what I want to be and I try to get on with
the task. Given the option, I would never have
chosen, and would not choose to repeat, this experience. Given the outcome, I regard it as one of
the richest episodes of my life. Because of the
losses I feared—life, social ease, love—and the
losses I felt—assurance of good health, confident
self-sufficiency, and a troublesome gland about
the size of a walnut—I am, and for some time will
be, more than I was.

THE PERSPECTIVE OF A PROSTATE CANCER DOCTOR

PETER T. SCARDINO, M.D.
Professor and Chairman
Scott Department of Urology
Baylor College of Medicine
Houston, Texas

When I began to practice medicine in the Texas Medical Center in 1979, I joined the National Prostate Cancer Project, an ambitious research program funded by the federal government and dedicated to discovering better treatment for advanced prostate cancer. It proved to be one of the most frustrating experiences of my professional life. Doctors from the leading medical centers in the country joined forces to try every available treatment that might slow the spread of the disease. Yet nothing we did altered the bleak outcome of our patients, with the modest exception of one study showing that a combination of hormone therapies (leuprolide plus flutamide) extended the survival of men with metastatic prostate cancer by about six months. No one was cured. Almost every man diagnosed with prostate cancer died of his disease.

This experience taught me a hard lesson: that our only hope in the foreseeable future of lowering the death rate from prostate cancer would be to detect the disease earlier, before it spread, and to eradicate it completely. In one of those great serendipitous occurrences that make a life in science so exciting, ten years of fruitless effort to find a cure for metastatic prostate cancer yielded instead a remarkable new test that would revolutionize early detection, the prostate specific antigen (PSA) test.

Although first discovered by Japanese scientists in the mid 1970s, it was not until the late 1980s that the power of this test came to be appreciated. Before PSA, seven of every ten cancers detected had spread beyond the point of cure. With PSA, seven of ten can be detected while still curable. Because the PSA level reflects the amount of prostate cancer in the body, PSA provides a powerful tool for monitoring the course of this cancer and the response to treatment. With PSA we can determine the success or failure of treatments rapidly, within four or five years, rather than waiting an agonizing ten or fifteen years.

Another major breakthrough in diagnosis occurred in the late 1980s. A simple way to see the prostate, by ultrasound imaging, was coupled with small, rapid-puncture biopsy needles that allowed multiple tissue samples to be taken from the prostate so that even small cancers could be detected. My practice changed dramatically. After years of disappointment and sadness over the inevitable deterioration of almost all my patients who had advanced prostate cancer, I now have the joy of seeing patients like Bill Martin, who return well, fully functional, with no trace of PSA, even many years after their treatment.

Still, prostate cancer remains a hotly debated topic, even among experts, and a source of confusion for many men struck with this disease.[1-4] Bill Martin asked me to write about the controversies, to spell out what we know about this disease now and what we need to learn if we are going to make progress against it. I hope the information presented here will be of some help to men faced with the tough choice of deciding what to do about their prostate cancer.

Not A Glamorous Topic

There is nothing glamorous about prostate cancer. In fact, there is nothing very glamorous about the prostate itself. Speaking to a ladies' luncheon about the prostate, as I occasionally do, is one of those experiences that almost makes me wish I were a *neurologist* rather than a *urologist*. But times are changing. This past year, feature stories on prostate cancer have run in the leading national news magazines, newspapers, and television news programs. World leaders, giants of industry, and celebrities—from Francois Mitterand, the President of France, to Michael Milken, the financier, to Jerry Lewis, the actor— have come forward to tell their stories. Quiet—even open— conversation about prostate cancer can be heard in retirement communities, golf courses, and board rooms around the country. In fact, wherever men over the age of 50 congregate, the prostate is likely to be a topic for discussion.

In spite of the well-deserved attention prostate cancer is finally getting, the message is mixed. Is this a serious disease or not? Should you worry about it? Should you be checked? Doesn't almost every man have a few cancer cells in his prostate anyway? Can a checkup really detect it? Should it be treated or left alone?

Some Disturbing Facts

Certainly prostate cancer is a frustrating and dangerous disease. There is no known cause and no way to prevent the disease. Diet and exercise

do not seem to help. A man can live by all the
rules, do all the right things, not smoke, eat a bal-
anced diet, get regular exercise, and still face a
slow, painful, protracted death from a cancer that
arises in an organ that he may never have heard
of. Prostate cancer is expected to affect 200,000
American men in 1994, and once it extends
beyond the prostate or immediate periprostatic
tissue, it cannot be cured. It is the most common
internal (non-skin) cancer in men in the Western
world and the second most common cause of cancer deaths. One man develops prostate cancer
every three minutes and one will die of the disease every fifteen minutes. It is the cause of death
in three of every 100 men. The incidence of this
disease rises faster with age than any other cancer.
As the average age of American men continues to
increase, the number of new cases each year is
expected to increase dramatically. Over the last
five years, the number of new cases doubled. As
other causes of death, such as cardiovascular disease, decline, the mortality rate from prostate cancer will continue to rise unless new techniques are
developed for prevention, early detection, or
treatment.

We do know something about risk factors for
prostate cancer. Age is the most powerful factor,
but race or ethnic background has a major influ-
ence. African American men have the highest

incidence in the world, much higher than native Africans. Men in northern European countries have the second highest incidence, while Asians uniformly have a very low risk of the disease.

It has only recently been accepted that prostate cancer can be a familial disease. As is the case for breast cancer, men who have either a brother or father—a "first-degree relative"—with prostate cancer, are 2-3 times more likely to develop the disease themselves; and if two first-degree relatives have it, risk is 8-11 times greater. Nearly half of all cases of prostate cancer in young men, under the age of 55, seem to be the familial variant, but this accounts for only about nine percent of all cases of prostate cancer. The gene can be passed from the mother's or the father's side.

Let's take a look at some other comparisons between prostate cancer and its closest cousin, breast cancer (Table 1). Both organs, the breast and the prostate, are under the control of the sex steroid hormones: the female hormone, estrogen, or the male hormone, androgen. In both cases, cancers of these organs can be influenced by changes in the circulating levels of these hormones. The numbers of new cases and deaths per year of prostate and breast cancer are similar, as is the ratio of deaths to new cases. The mortality rates of both diseases have been increasing steadily, even when the aging of the population is taken

Table 1.

Similarities of Breast and Prostate Cancer

	Breast Cancer	Prostate Cancer
New cases/yr	182,000	200,000
Deaths/yr	46,000	38,000
Ratio deaths/cases	25.3%	19.0%
Trends in mortality rates (30 yr)	Increasing: 6%	Increasing 17%
Median age at:		
Diagnosis	64	71
Death	66	77
Five-year survival rate:		
All Stages	79%	77%
Localized	93%	92%
Regional	73%	82%
Metastatic	19%	29%
Stage at diagnosis:		
Localized	53%	58%
Regional	37%	14%
Metastatic	7%	18%

into consideration. This means that both diseases are taking a greater toll in lives. The median ages at diagnosis of and death from prostate cancer are a bit higher than for breast cancer, but it is a common misconception that breast cancer usually strikes young women in their prime, while prostate cancer only strikes elderly men. The relative survival rates at five years are almost identical and the stage (or extent) of the disease at the time of diagnosis is quite similar. In fact, with the availability of PSA, even fewer men have metastases at the time of diagnosis of prostate cancer, so the stage at diagnosis is likely to become virtually identical.

Why The Controversy?

The controversy and confusion about prostate cancer arise from several unique features of this disease which make it a bit different from any other cancer. In the first place, prostate cancer is slow growing. Its doubling time, when still localized within the prostate, has been estimated at 2-4 years. There certainly are men with prostate cancer who live out their lives without any effects from the disease. When small foci of well differentiated cancer are detected incidentally in prostatic tissue removed to relieve urinary obstruction, the disease poses little risk to life or health, and there is a general consensus that most men with cancer of this type (T1a) do not need to be treated, but simply followed with a checkup from time to time. In the Scandinavian countries and Great Britain, there has been a general policy of "benign neglect" towards this disease. "Watchful waiting" is the favored management strategy, and few men with well or moderately differentiated cancers that are causing no symptoms and are located within the prostate die of their cancer within 10 years.[5-7]

A second reason for the confusion arises from the relatively elderly population of men diagnosed with prostate cancer. Many of these men are in an age group when death from other causes becomes statistically probable within 10 years. In 1989, a median life expectancy of 10 years occurred at age 73.6. Since relatively few men with early prostate cancer will die of their disease within 10 years, and the median age of diagnosis is 71 years, and since the growth of the tumor can be slowed markedly by relatively simple hormonal manipulation, a man may face little threat from this slow-growing tumor if his age or health indicate a life expectancy less than 10 years.

But the feature that really makes prostate cancer unique, and thoroughly confuses the novice, is that cancer cells can be found within the prostate in over one-third of all men over the age of 50.

(This figure has been confirmed repeatedly by reports of the presence of microscopic cancer cells detected during autopsy.) Since more than 30 million American men are over the age of 50, this stark statistic means that over 10 million men in this country have prostate cancer right now. Detecting 200,000 new patients per year seems like sighting the tip of the iceberg. Since prostate cancer grows so slowly, I have found it easier to understand the relationship between this type of microscopic cancer, found so frequently in the prostates of otherwise perfectly healthy men, and a truly health- and life-threatening form of prostate cancer, by analyzing the lifetime risk that a 50-year-old man will develop one of these forms of prostate cancer. Statistically, over the lifetime of men now 50 years old, 42 of every 100 will develop cancer in the prostate, ten will actually be diagnosed with prostate cancer, and three will die of the disease.[8] These figures tell us clearly that not every prostate cancer needs to be detected and treated—only those that pose a threat to life or health.

The final reason for the controversy is that there is no definitive proof that would convince a hardened skeptic that early detection or treatment of prostate cancer will lower the chances of dying from this disease. It is not that good studies have failed to prove that treatment is beneficial. The studies have simply not been done. The absence of evidence, however, should not be construed as evidence of absence. Detecting prostate cancer early and treating it while it can still be cured may well be the only effective strategy we have for lowering the death rate from this disease. But we do not know for sure.

The studies have not been done because prostate cancer has been the poor stepchild of our otherwise enormously successful medical research enterprise. As just one example, the National Institutes of Health provided nearly $200 million for research on breast cancer in 1993, or approximately $4,300 for every death from breast cancer the previous year. In contrast, only $36 million was available to support research in prostate cancer, or $1,100 for every death. A few years ago I could count the number of full-time physicians or scientists who devote their lives to the study of prostate cancer on the fingers of two hands. With such limited effort, there is too little information.

The Good News

With increasing public awareness of the disease, and with the attention that prostate cancer has garnered through the courageous efforts of highly visible public figures, such as Senator Robert Dole, the tide has begun to change.

Funding through the National Cancer Institute is increasing, though it still lags far behind that for breast cancer and AIDS. Research is expanding. Two years ago Specialized Programs of Research Excellence (SPOREs) in Prostate Cancer were created by the National Cancer Institute, one at the Baylor College of Medicine in Houston and the other at the Johns Hopkins Hospital in Baltimore. Funds have been committed for the most important long-term clinical studies to determine 1) whether screening for prostate cancer with PSA and the digital rectal examination (DRE) will lower the death rate from this disease (the "PLCO" trial), 2) whether treatment is superior to watchful waiting for men with localized prostate cancer (the "PIVOT" trial), and 3) whether prostate cancer can be prevented by the use of finasteride (the "Prevention" trial). Finasteride is a new drug produced by Merck and Company under the brand name Proscar, and was originally designed for the treatment of benign enlargement of the prostate (BPH).

Early Detection

The major limitation in the treatment of prostate cancer in the past was our inability to detect the disease before it spread. Since prostate cancer typically causes no symptoms in it early stages, and since it is incurable in its advanced stages, there was a desperate need for a sensitive new diagnostic test. Even when men came for the traditional yearly DRE, seven of every ten cancers had already spread when first detected.[8,9] PSA revolutionized the early detection of this disease. PSA combined with DRE nearly doubled the detection rate compared to detection by DRE alone. Recent studies have confirmed the remarkable performance capabilities of PSA. In the most widely used assay, a PSA level greater than 4.0 ng/ml is considered abnormal. If the PSA was greater than four, cancer was found in nearly one-third of men.[10]   The higher the PSA, the greater the chances a cancer would be found when a needle biopsy of the prostate was done. And most remarkably, when PSA was used in combination with DRE, 70 percent of the cancers detected were still confined to the prostate glands when they were removed surgically, compared to only 30 percent before the PSA era. It is not hard to understand why the American Cancer Society and the American Urological Association recommend a DRE and PSA test annually in healthy men over the age of 50 with a life expectancy greater than ten years and in men over the age of 40 who are at increased risk of prostate cancer—for example, men of African-American descent or those with a family history of the disease. Nevertheless, we must recognize that no studies have been done to prove definitively that screening for prostate cancer with any test, whether the DRE or PSA, will lower the risk that a man will die from this disease.

Concern has been raised about the seriousness of cancers detected with the PSA test. *Time* magazine reflected this concern, asking whether the PSA test "may be turning up the less troublesome tumors and not ferreting out the killer cancers."[11] The answer: not true. Cancers detected by PSA are 50-100 times larger, 5-6 times more likely to be poorly differentiated (high Gleason grade), and 15-20 times more likely to extend outside of the prostate than the indolent cancers found in a third of men over the age of 50.[12,13] The level of the PSA in the blood generally correlates well with the size of a prostate cancer, so it requires a cancer of at least 1 gram to produce a PSA level above normal. When cancers of this size double 2-3 times, over 4-6 years, they advance from a small cancer that can easily be cured with surgery to one that has spread beyond the prostate and can rarely be cured.

Recently, a number of attempts have been made to increase the performance and usefulness of the PSA test. For example *age-specific adjustments* of the normal range—lowering the cutoff to 2.5 ng/ml for men in their forties, 3.5 ng/ml for men in their fifties, 4.5 ng/ml for men in their

sixties, and 6.5 ng/ml for men in their seventies—
might allow more cancers to be detected in
younger men, while decreasing the number of
older men recommended for a biopsy because
their PSA is elevated.[14] PSA *density* corrects the
PSA level for the size of the prostate (measured by
ultrasound). Since PSA is produced by normal
prostatic tissue as well as by cancer, as the
prostate grows larger with BPH, the PSA level
may increase as well. But cancer releases ten
times as much PSA into the circulation, per gram
of tissue, as does BPH. A high PSA density (a
PSA level too high for the size of the prostate)
may therefore signal the presence of cancer.[15]
Others have focused on PSA *velocity*, or the rate of
change in the PSA level over time, finding that if
the level rises more than 0.75 ng/ml per year, the
chances of finding cancer are increased [16]
Nevertheless, none of these modifications have
proven to be more practical, efficient, or effective
in detecting cancer or avoiding unnecessary biopsies than the use of the standard PSA test.

There are some pitfalls in interpreting PSA
results. Not all laboratory assays are the same.
The results are not necessarily comparable from
one laboratory to another. PSA is not cancer-
specific, but prostate-specific. The levels rise as
the prostate enlarges with benign prostatic hyperplasia (BPH) and can increase dramatically during

episodes of infection (prostatitis) or following trauma to the prostate, such as with a needle biopsy or a prostate resection. A finger examination of the prostate, however, does not alter the PSA level appreciably. No other disease produces a steady continuous rise in the PSA level over many months except cancer.

An elevated PSA test does not prove that a man has prostate cancer. Rather, it indicates the need for further testing, which usually involves an ultrasonic examination of the prostate gland and an ultrasound-guided needle biopsy. Generally, biopsies would be recommended for any man who is a candidate for definitive therapy; that is, any man whose age and overall health are consistent with a life expectancy of at least 8-10 years, and who would find the risk of treatment acceptable.

One of the most spectacular successes of the PSA test is its ability to signal the results of treatment many years before traditional tests, such as the bone scan, serum acid phosphatase level, or even a medical history and physical examination. If the prostate is completely removed during a radical prostatectomy, the PSA level should fall and become undetectable. A measurable and rising PSA level after radical prostatectomy or irradiation therapy invariably means that the cancer is still present and growing, although a normal or undetectable level does not necessarily prove that the cancer has been cured. There is no better measure of the success or failure of treatment of prostate cancer than the serum PSA level. We have found in our own patient population that it is rare for a patient ever to develop an elevated PSA level if it remains undetectable for the first five years after radical prostatectomy.

Treatment

One of the most difficult decisions facing a man diagnosed with prostate cancer is whether to be treated with surgery or radiation therapy — or to receive no treatment at all. The scientific information is simply not available to tell with certainty which treatment is the best. Men who have prostate cancer have to make a decision, together with their physicians, on the basis of the available evidence. While we do not know which treatment is "the best" for every person, we do have a great deal of information that can help each man make a reasonable choice about what is best for him. Although many treatments have been used for localized prostate cancer — such as implantation of radioactive seeds into the prostate, cryosurgery (freezing), and "neoadjuvant" hormonal therapy combined with surgery — I would like to address the most commonly used and time-honored treatments, radical prostatectomy and radiotherapy, as

well as the major reasonable alternative, "watchful waiting."

Radical Prostatectomy

Radical prostatectomy, the total removal of the
prostate and seminal vesicles, was developed
early in this century and continues to be improved
today. The major advantage of this operation is
the confidence we have in the long-term cure of
the cancer. Studies of patients followed for as
long as 25-30 years have shown that radical
prostatectomy can result in lifelong freedom from
cancer in a substantial proportion of men.[17,18] In
our experience at Baylor with over 500 patients
with localized prostate cancer (clinical stage T1-2)
followed for 1-11 years after the operation, 80 percent have no evidence of recurrence of their cancer and have an undetectable PSA level at 5 years,
and 76 percent are free of cancer at 10 years.
Today radical prostatectomy can be performed
with a high degree of safety. The chances of a serious complication are low; for example, pneumo-
nia, thrombophlebitis, pulmonary embolism, or
myocardial infarctions occur in fewer than 2-3
percent of men. Blood transfusions are rarely necessary. At The Methodist Hospital in Houston,
where I work, we no longer ask patients to place
their own blood in the blood bank (autologous
donation), and the need for a blood transfusion is

less than one in 25 patients. A fatal complication from the operation occurs in 1-2 patients for every 1,000 operated upon in major medical centers by expert surgeons. Most men are out of the hospital within 4-5 days and will regain normal urinary control within weeks or months. The chances of severe and permanent urinary incontinence are now 1-2 percent in the hands of highly experienced surgeons. In our series, 94 percent of men have regained normal urinary control at one year, 4-5 percent had mild stress urinary incontinence, and one percent had severe incontinence. Urinary incontinence is age related and is quite rare in men under the age of 60. Penile erections were once impossible to preserve after this operation,[19] but today, in many men with early tumors confined to the prostate gland, the neurovascular bundles that regulate erections can be preserved, and erections will return within months. The risk of impotence varies with the location and the extent of the tumor, the quality of erections before the operation, and the skill and experience of the surgeon in identifying and preserving the neurovascular bundles. While both incontinence and impotence are serious problems, neither is life-threatening and both can be successfully treated, so very few men are faced with living the rest of their lives disabled by the lack of satisfactory urinary or sexual function.

Certainly, the major disadvantages of a radical prostatectomy are the need for hospitalization, the risks of a major surgical procedure, and the expense. In general, the risks of this operation for a man are similar to the risks of a hysterectomy for a woman. There is time lost from work (usually 3-6 weeks) and the inconvenience and anguish of temporary urinary and sexual dysfunction.

Radiation Therapy

Radiotherapy is administered with high-dose linear accelerators (at least 15 MeV, which means at least 15 million electron volts) and can now be done with considerable safety. Using computerized tomography (CT or "cat") scans to localize the prostate precisely, and highly sophisticated techniques for shielding the normal tissue, the risk of complications from external beam radiation therapy has diminished markedly over the last two decades. While once there were strong reasons to search for alternatives for external beam therapy, because of the damaging effects on the rectum and urinary bladder that lie so close to the prostate, recent studies have shown no advantage in safety or effectiveness for other forms of radiation, such as radioactive seed implantation.

Radiation therapy is administered daily, usually Monday through Friday, over a period of seven weeks. The side effects are cumulative, with the most common being diarrhea, which can usually be controlled with oral medications and disappears within a few months. Only 1-3 percent of men will have long-term problems with proctitis (inflammation of the rectum) for months or years following radiation therapy.

The major advantage of radiation therapy, of course, is that no operation or hospitalization is necessary. Many men find that they can continue to perform most of their regular activities while receiving radiation therapy. There is less time lost from work and other activities with radiation therapy than with radical prostatectomy. Radiation therapy itself rarely, if ever, causes urinary incontinence, although, if the cancer is not eradicated, urinary incontinence can arise in the future with additional efforts to control the local tumor. Impotence, which can occur, seems to be less common than after radical prostatectomy and to develop more slowly. In the largest study reported, half of the men lost their erections by seven years after radiation therapy.[20] All in all, radiotherapy is easier to go through than radical prostatectomy.

The major disadvantage of radiotherapy is the difficulty in eradicating the cancer completely. While this is a highly controversial subject, a disturbing percentage of men treated with radiotherapy will still have cancer cells present in the prostate 2-3 years later if a needle biopsy is done. The PSA level almost always drops steadily after radiotherapy, but begins to rise again within several years in some patients. In recent reports, about 40-55 percent of men with localized prostate cancer (clinical stage T1-2) will begin to experience a rise in their PSA levels by five years after radiotherapy. It is difficult to be certain whether the tumor has been completely eradicated after radiotherapy, and it is uncertain what could be done if it has not been. Further attempts at cure, such as salvage radical prostatectomy, are difficult after radiotherapy, and no treatment is widely accepted as safe and effective.[21]

Brachytherapy with radioactive seed implants is less popular now because of the technical difficulty in placing the seeds accurately and in assuring a uniform dose to the entire cancer. Seed implants usually require hospitalization and anesthesia, the rate of local recurrence is high, and the lack of sufficient data to judge the effectiveness and the complication rate of new methods involving ultrasound-guided implantations with palladium or iodine seeds make these treatments chancy.

For these reasons, it is generally recommended that young men with small cancers confined to the prostate are better treated with radical prostatectomy, while older men, or those with health problems that would make an operation risky, and those with large tumors that are unlikely to be removed completely by surgery, are best treated with radiation therapy. Both forms of treatment have stood the test of time, both are potentially curative, and both are widely used throughout the country, so that a patient would have a choice of many experienced physicians. Making a choice between these treatments is something that each man must decide for himself, in consultation with his physician, after careful consideration of the advantages and disadvantages of each.[22]

Watchful Waiting

An alternative strategy for the treatment of localized prostate cancer is *watchful waiting*. This approach has recently received considerable attention, particularly in the Scandinavian countries and Great Britain, where studies are underway to try to establish the risk of leaving a localized prostate cancer untreated.[5,7,23,24] Most patients included in these studies are older, have very small, well-differentiated cancers (clinical stage T1a), and other problems with their health that limit their expected survival. These men have been judged by the physician to be more likely to die of other causes than of their prostate cancer. While watchful waiting has received less publicity in the United States, it is actually widely used. A

survey conducted by the American College of
Surgeons showed that "no treatment" was the
most common initial approach recommended by
physicians for patients diagnosed with prostate
cancer.[25] All of us have patients who, because of
their age, their general health, or because they
have a small, extremely favorable tumor, are best
treated with a watchful waiting approach. In my
own practice, I have recommended radical prostatectomy for 85 percent of the patients referred to
me, radiation therapy for ten percent, and watchful waiting for five percent. Today, with PSA levels available and with the ease of ultrasound-
guided needle biopsy of the prostate, it is much
more feasible to follow the course of cancer in
carefully selected men and defer their further
treatment until there is a clear sign that the cancer
is progressing. The danger with this approach, of
course, is that the cancer could spread and
become incurable *while it is being watched.*

In a widely quoted 1993 medical report, the
Prostate Patient Outcomes Research Team (PORT)
published a computerized decision-analysis
model of the treatment of localized prostate cancer.[26] Based upon the best information they could
glean from the published medical literature, they
analyzed the benefit, in quality-adjusted life years
added, from definitive treatment of prostate cancer with radical prostatectomy or radiation therapy

compared to a watchful waiting approach. The PORT model assumed that the most common form of prostate cancer, a moderately-differentiated tumor, presented a 1.3 percent risk of metastasizing per year if left untreated. At this slow rate of spread, they calculated that the average 65-year-old man would gain only 0.33 quality-adjusted life years by active treatment. They concluded that treatment offered only marginal benefit when the age and life expectancy of the patient and the risk of the treatment itself were taken into consideration.

A group from Baylor recently analyzed this model, confirming that the most important determinant of the amount of benefit gained by treatment was the rate at which prostate cancer was assumed to metastasize each year the patient was in a watchful waiting program. In this analysis, the chances that a moderately-differentiated cancer would metastasize each year were 4.2 *times greater* than the highest rate estimated by the PORT group. At this rate, the benefit of treating a 65-year-old man with a well-differentiated tumor increased from 0.33 to 2.41 quality-adjusted life years.[27] Computer modeling is one way of estimating the benefit of treatment based upon the available information, but firm proof of the benefits of treatment must await a controlled clinical trial comparing active treatment with watchful waiting.[28,29]

We have learned a great deal about prostate cancer in the past ten years. The next decade will see an explosion of new knowledge about this far-too-common disease. PSA has proved to be the best cancer marker known to medicine and a highly sensitive monitor of the outcome of treatment. The PSA level before treatment is the best single predictor of prognosis. We now know that surgery frequently can cure prostate cancer when the cancer is confined within the prostate gland itself, but rarely is able to cure the disease when it has spread to adjacent structures such as seminal vesicles or pelvic lymph nodes. While radiotherapy can control prostate cancer for long periods in some patients, PSA levels show that the cancer will begin to recur in a disturbing proportion of these patients within a few years. Even with radical prostatectomy, PSA levels eventually rise in 25-30 percent of patients, demonstrating the difficulty we still have in controlling prostate cancer when there is even microscopic spread beyond the immediate area of the prostate itself.

Unfortunately, no valid randomized study has been completed that could demonstrate which treatment is best for patients with clinically localized prostate cancer, or whether any treatment is better than watchful waiting. Fortunately, several trials are underway and answers may come within the next 10-15 years.[29,30] Until then, research

will focus on new tests that will allow us to estimate, in each patient with prostate cancer, the
degree of danger that the cancer poses so that the
treatment used is appropriate to the threat of the
disease itself. Until that time arrives, men found
to have a localized prostate cancer should, with
the help of their physicians, develop a clear
understanding of the nature of their cancer and
the risk it poses, honestly estimate their life
expectancy based on their age, general health, and
family history, and then examine the available
treatment options in light of their own values.
With a thorough understanding of the advantages
and disadvantages of each treatment alternative, a
man afflicted with this far-too-common cancer can
make a decision with which he can feel comfortable, as Bill Martin did, and will be blessed with
the good fortune of the wonderful outcome that
Bill describes in this chronicle of his own experience with the leading cancer in American men.

References

[1]Alexander, T. One man's tough choices on prostate
cancer. *Fortune*, September 20, 1993, pp. 86-98.

[2]Eddy, D.M. Three battles to watch in the 1990s.
Clinical Decision Making: From Theory to Practice.
Journal of the American Medical Association (JAMA)
270:520-526, 1993.

[3]Garnick, M. The dilemmas of prostate cancer:

Scientific American, April, 1994, pp. 72-81.

[4]Mann, C.C. The prostate-cancer dilemma. *The Atlantic Monthly*, November, 1993, pp. 102-118.

[5]Adolfsson, J., Carstensen, J. Natural course of clinically localized prostate adenocarcinoma in men less than 70 years old. *Journal of Urology*. 146: 96, 1991.

[6]George, N.J. Conservative management of prostate cancer: Letter. *Lancet* 1: 1001, 1988.

[7]Johansson, J.E., Adami, H.O., Andersson, S.O., Bergstrom, R., Holberg, L. and Krusemo, U.B. High 10-year survival rate in patients with early, untreated prostatic cancer. *JAMA* 269:2650-9, 1993.

[8]Scardino, P.T., Weaver, R., and Hudson, M.A. Early detection of prostate cancer. *Human Pathology* 23: 211, 1992.

[9]Gerber, G.S., Thompson , I.M., Thisted, R. .Chodak, G.W. Disease-specific survival following routine prostate cancer screening by digital rectal examination. *JAMA* 269: 61-64, 1993.

[10]Catalona, W.J., Richie, J.P., Ahmann, F.R., Hudson, M.A., Scardino, P.T., Flanigan, R.C., deKernion, J.B., Ratliff, T.L., Kavoussi, L.R., Dalkin, B.L., Waters, W.B., MacFarlane, M.T., and Southwick, P.C. Comparison of digital rectal examination and serum prostate specific antigen in the early detection of prostate cancer: Results of a multicenter clinical trial of 6,630 men. *Journal of Urology* 151: 1283, 1994.

[11]Gorman, C. The private pain of prostate cancer. *Time*, October 5, 1992, p.77.

[12]Ohori, M., Wheeler, T.M., and Scardino, P.T. The pathologic features and prognosis of prostate cancers detectable with current diagnostic tests. *Journal of Urology* Supplement, 1994.

[13]Ohori, M., Wheeler, T.M., and Scardino, P.T. The new American Joint Committee on Cancer and International Union Against Cancer TNM classification of prostate cancer: Clinicopathologic correlations. *Cancer* 74: 104-114, 1994.

[14]Oesterling, J.E., Jacobsen, S.J., Chute, C.G., Guess, H.A., Girman, C.J., Panser, L.A., and Lieber, M.M. Serum prostate-specific antigen in a community-based population of healthy men: Establishment of age-specific reference ranges. *JAMA* 270: 860, 1993.

[15]Benson, M.D., Whang, I.S., Olsson, C.A., McMahon, D.J., Cooner, W.H. The use of prostate specific antigen density to enhance the predictive value of intermediate levels of serum prostate specific antigen. *Journal of Urology* 147:817, 1992.

[16]Carter, H.B., Pearson, J.D., Metter, E.J., Brant, L.J., Chan, D.W., Andres, R., Fozard, J.L., and Walsh, P.C. Longitudinal evaluation of prostate-specific antigen levels in men with and without prostate disease. *JAMA* 267: 2215, 1992.

[17]Gibbons, R.P., Correa, R.J., Jr., Brannen, G.E., Weissman, R.M. Total prostatectomy for clinically localized prostatic cancer: Long-term results. *Journal of Urology* 141:564, 1989.

[18]Lepor, H., Kimball, A.W., Walsh, P.C. Cause-

specific actuarial survival analysis: A useful method for reporting survival data in men with clinically localized carcinoma of the prostate. *Journal of Urology* 141: 82, 1989.

[19]Walsh P.C. and Donker, P.J. Impotence following radical prostatectomy: Insight into etiology and prevention. *Journal of Urology* 128:492, 1982.

[20]Goffinet, D., Bagshaw, M.A. Radiation therapy of prostate cancer. In: Crawford, E.D., Das, S. eds. *Current Genitourinary Surgery*. Philadelphia: Lea & Febiger, 1990, p. 552.

[21]Rogers, E., Ohori, M., Kassabian, V.S., Wheeler, T.M., and Scardino, P.T. Salvage radical prostatectomy: Outcome measured by serum prostate specific antigen levels. (Submitted, 1994).

[22]National Institutes of Health Consensus Development Panel: Consensus statement. The management of clinically localized prostate cancer. *National Cancer Institute Monographs* 7: 3, 1988.

[23]Adolfsson, J., Carstensen, J., and Lowhagen, T. Deferred treatment in clinically localized prostatic carcinoma. *British Journal of Urology*. 69:183, 1992.

[24]Chodak G.W., Thisted, R.A., Gerber, G.S. et al. Results of conservative management of clinically localized prostate cancer. *New England Journal of Medicine* 330:242-248, 1994.

[25]Mettlin, C., Jones, G.W., Murphy, G.P. Trends in prostate cancer care in the United States, 1974-1990: Observations from the patient care evaluation studies

of the American College of Surgeons Commission on Cancer. *CA-A Cancer Journal for Clinicians* 43:83, 1993.

[26]Fleming, C., Wasson J.H., Albertsen, P.C., Barry, M.J., Wennberg, J.E. for the Prostate PORT. A decision analysis of alternative treatment strategies for clinically localized prostate cancer. *JAMA* 269:2650, 1993.

[27]Scardino, P.T., Beck, J.R., Miles, B.J. Conservative management of prostate cancer: Letter to the Editor. *New England Journal of Medicine* 330:1831, 1994.

[28]Beck, J.R., Kattan, M.W., and Miles, B.J. A critique of the decision anaysis for clinically localized prostate cancer. *Journal of Urology* Supplement, 1994.

[29]Wilt, T.J., and Brawer, M.K. The Prostate Cancer Intervention Versus Observation trial (PIVOT) A randomized trial comparing radical prostatectomy versus expectant management for the treatment of clinically localized prostate cancer. *Journal of Urology* Supplement, 1994.

[30]Gohagan, J.K., Prorok, P.C., Kramer, B.S., Cornett, J.E. Prostate cancer screening in the prostate, lung, colorectal, and ovarian cancer screening trial of the national cancer institute. *Journal of Urology* Supplement, 1994.

NOTES

[1]"1.7 million doctor visits." Sandra Salsmans, *Prostate: Questions You Have...Answers You Need* (Allentown, PA: People's Medical Society, 1993), pp. 39-41.

[2]gland "causes more misery." Ibid., p. 16.

[3]"[TURP] must be learned with painstaking care." A. Walsh, "Indications for prostatic surgery and selection of operation," in John M. Fitzpatrick and Robert J. Krane, *The Prostate* (Edinburgh: Churchill Livingstone, 1989), pp. 137-142 F/K, p. 140.

[4]"anyone under sixty-five as young." Tom Alexander, "One Man's Tough Choices on Prostate Cancer," *Fortune*, September 20, 1993, pp. 86-10.

[5]"environmental factors must play a key role." Frank P. Begun, "Epidemiology and Natural History of Prostate Cancer," in Herbert Lepor, MD, and Russell K. Lawson, MD., *Prostate Diseases* (Philadelphhia: W. B. Saunders Company, 1993) p. 258.

[6]Varying rates of prostate cancer. Ibid., pp. 255-256.

[7]Prostate cancer in African-Americans. B. Lytton, "Demography of prostatic carcinoma," in Fitzpatrick and Krane, *The Prostate*, pp. 254-256.

[8]Diet and prostate cancer. Begun, pp. 259-260; Salmans, p. 85.

[9]Occupation and prostate cancer. Begun, p. 259; Salmans, p. 87.

[10]Vasectomy and prostate cancer. Salmans, p. 60.

[11]The role of heredity. Ibid, p. 63, citing National Cancer Institute data.

[12]Senator Dole: "be on the lookout." Ibid., p. 62.

[13]"eunuchs don't get prostate cancer." Begun, p. 260.

[14]Stamey's hypothesis. Begun, pp. 261-262.

[15]Whitmore's question. Ibid. Also, W. F. Whitmore, Jr., "Natural History of low-stage prostatic cancer and the impact of early detection," *Urologic Clinics of North America* 17:689, 1990; Thomas Stamey, "Cancer of the Prostate: An Analysis of Some Important Contributions and Dilemmas," *Monographs in Urology* 3:67, 1982. Also, cited by Begun, J. E. McNeal, D. G. Bostwick, R. A. Kindrachuk, et al. "Patterns of progression in prostate cancer." *Lancet* 1:60, 1986.

[16]PSA scores. M. C. Benson and C. A. Olsson, "The Staging and Grading of Prostatic Cancer," Fitzpatrick and Krane, *The Prostate*, p. 267.

[17]Variation on Gleason scoring. Ibid.

[18]Staging and grading of prostate cancers. Stephen Rous, *The Prostate Book: Sound Advice on Symptoms and Treatment* (New York: W. W. Norton, 1988), pp. 136-138; Benson and Olsson, op. cit., pp. 265-266; R. K. Babayan, "Diagnosis and methods of staging prostatic carcinoma," Fitzpatrick and Krane, *The Prostate*, pp. 273-280.

[19]The TNM Classification system. M. C. Benson, C. A. Olsson, op. cit., p. 265-267; F. K. Mostofi, Charles J. Davis, Jr., and Isabell A. Sesterhenn, "Histopathology of

Prostate Cancer" Lepor and Lawson, *Prostate Diseuses*, p. 239; Makoto Ohori MD, Thomas M. Wheeler MD, and Peter T. Scardino MD, "The new TNM classification of PC: Clinicopathologic correlations." Manuscript in progress.

[20]Risks of radiation therapy. W. J. Taylor, "Radiation oncology: cancer of the prostate," *Cancer* 39: 856; J. S. Mollenkamp , J. F. Cooper , A. R. Kagen, "Clinical experience with supervoltage readiotherapy in carcinoma of the P: A prelim. report," *Journal of Urology*, 133:374, 1975; M. A. Bagshaw, "Definitive megavoltage radiation therapy in caracinoma of the prostate," In G. H. Fletch (ed), *Textbook of Radiotherapy* (Philadelphia: Lea and Febiger, 1973), pp. 752-767; M. A. Bagshaw, R. G. Ray, D. A. Pistenna, "External beam radiation therapy for primary carcinoma of the prostate," *Cancer* 36 (1975), p. 723 ; R. K. Rhamy, S. K. Wilson, W. I. Caldwell, "Biopsy proved tumor following definite irradiation for esectable carcinoma of the prostate," *Journal of Urology* 107 (1972), p. 627; G. R. Ray, J. R. Cassady, M. A. Bagshaw, "Definitive Radiotherapy of Carcinoma of the Prostate," *Therapeutic Radiotherapy*, 106 (1973), p. 407.

[21]Deaths from prostate surgery. Marc B. Garnick, "The Dilemmas of Prostate Cancer," *Scientific American* (April 1994), p. 78.

[22]Radiation therapy. M. A. Bagshaw, "The managment of prostatic carcinoma by radiotherapy," Fitzpatrick and Krane, *The Prostate*, pp. 359-375.

[23]"no evidence the average urologist performs..." Barry E. Epstein and Gerald E. Hanks, "Prostate Cancer: Evaluation and Radiotherapeutic Management," *CA-A Cancer Journal for Clinicians* 42:4 (July/August 1992), p 235; also, C. Eggleston and P. C. Walsh, "Radical Prostatectomy with preservation of sexual function: pathological findings in the first 100 cases. *Journal of Urology*, 134:1149; P. C. Walsh, H. Lepor, J. C. Eggleston, "Radical Prostatectomy with preservation of sexual function: anatomical and pathological considerations," *Prostate* 4:473; William J. Catalona and S. M. Dresner, "Nerve-sparing radical prostatectomy: extraprostatic tumor extension and prevention of erectile failure." *Journal of Urology* 134: 1149 (1985); A. L. Finkle and R. O. Williams, "Sexual potency before and after radical prostatectomy," *Western Journal of Medicine* 143:474.

[24]"Walsh observed, to his excitement." Charles C. Mann, "The Prostate Cancer Dilemma," *The Atlantic Monthly*, November 1993, p. 115.

[25]"a death of rare awfulness." Ibid.

[26]"the best surgeon I could find." Ibid., p. 118.

[27]"we've got a 95 percent chance." As optimistic as this sounds, it is actually a conservative estimate. At the beginning of 1994, no patient whose T1c tumor Scardino had removed had experienced a recurrence of his cancer.

APPENDIX

A COMPARISON OF STAGING SYSTEMS
FOR PROSTATE CANCER

WHITEMORE-JEWETT
(ABCD System)

Stage A.
Tumor undetectable by DRE or TRUS.

A1. Tumor occupies less than 5 percent of tissue specimen, and is well-differentiated.

A2. Tumor occupies more than 5 percent of tissue specimen and is moderately or poorly differ-·entiated.

Stage B.
Tumor detectable by DRE, but confined within the prostate.

B1. Single nodule, no larger than two centimeters, confined to one lobe (zone).

B2. More than one nodule or larger than 2 cm, but confined to prostate.

B3. Tumor involves both lobes.

Stage C.
Tumors larger, extend through the prostate capsule, with no evidence of metastasis.

C1. Tumor smaller than 6 cm. in diameter.

C2. Tumor larger than 6 cm. in diameter.

TNM SYSTEM

Tumor Status:

T-Zero.
No evidence of primary tumor.

T1. Tumor undetectable by DRE or TRUS.

T1a. Tumor an incidental finding in 5 percent or less of tissue removed in treatment of BPH.

T1b. Tumor an incidental finding in more than 5 percent tissue removed in treatment of BPH.

T1c. Tumor identified by needle biopsy, usually taken because of elevated serum PSA.

T2.
Tumor detectable by DRE or TRUS, but confined within the prostate.

T2a. Tumor involves half of one lobe (zone) or less.

T2b. Tumor involves more than half of one lobe, but not both lobes.

T2c. Tumor involves both lobes.

T3.
Tumor extends through the prostate capsule.

T3a. Extension through only one side of capsule.

T3b. Extension through both sides.

T3c. Extension into seminal vesicles.

245

Stage D.

Tumor has spread (metastasized) beyond the seminal vesicles.

D1. Tumor invades lymph nodes, but not beyond.

D2. Tumor has spread beyond lymph nodes to organs and/or bones.

T4.

Tumor invades adjacent structures other than the seminal vesicles.

T4a. Extension to bladder neck and/or external sphincter and/or rectum.

T4b. Tumor invades surrounding muscles and/or is fixed to the pelvic wall.

Nodal Status

N-X and N-zero. Lymph nodes are not assessed (X) or not involved (zero).

N1. Cancer extends to one node, in the immediate region of the prostate.

N2. Multiple nodes involved.

N3. Involvement of fixed nodal mass not attached to the tumor.

N4. Cancer extends to nodes in other regions of the body.

Metastatic Status

M-X and M-zero. Metastasis not assessed (X) or not present (zero).

M1a. Biochemical evidence of metastasis.

M1b. Single metastasis in single organ site (e.g., liver or lungs).

M3c. Multiple metastasis in single site.

M1d. Multiple metastatic sites.

WILLIAM MARTIN, Professor of Sociology at Rice University, is the author of four earlier books and more than a hundred articles, most of which have appeared in such magazines as *The Atlantic Monthly, Esquire Harper's,* and *Texas Monthly.* His biography, *A Prophet with Honor: The Billy Graham Story,* was published in 1991 by William Morrow and Company.

PETER T. SCARDINO, M.D. is Chairman of the Scott Department of Urology at Baylor College of Medicine in Houston. In 1992, he was appointed principal investigator for the Specialized Programs of Research Excellence made possible by a National Institutes of Health grant to foster new ways to diagnose, prevent, and treat prostate cancer. He currently serves as Chairman of the Prostate Health Council of the American Foundation of Urologic Disease.